Detox

Your Diet

A 28-Day Detox Plan

How to Banish Addictive Foods, Lose Weight Naturally & Send Your Energy Levels Through the Roof!

Lise Cartwright

www.detoxyourdietplan.com

ISBN-13: 978-1545062258
ISBN-10: 1545062250

Disclaimer

The information provided in this book is presented for educational purposes only and should not be used in lieu of advice from your doctor or qualified healthcare provider. Results from the use of Arbonne and other products mentioned, vary depending upon individual effort, body composition, age, eating patterns, and exercise. If you have a medical condition or are pregnant or breastfeeding, the author recommends that you consult with your healthcare professional before starting any type of healthcare regimen, including the detox plan outlined in this book.

The author accepts no responsibility for any injury or health complications resulting from the reader using the educational information provided within this book. If in doubt, please seek advice from your doctor or healthcare professional.

DOWNLOAD THE
COMPANION ACTION GUIDE!

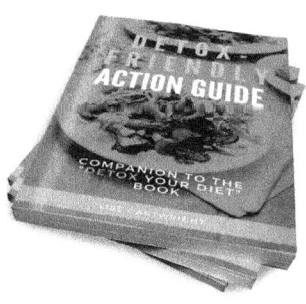

READ THIS FIRST

I've found that readers get the most success with this book when they use the **Detox Friendly Action Guide** as they read along.

And just to say thanks for buying my book, I'd love to give you access to the ***Detox Friendly Action Guide for FREE***.

Visit www.detoxyourdietplan.com/free-gift

Dedication

This book is dedicated to my amazing friend, Sammy D, who continues to inspire and push me to greater heights.

Thank you :-)

Acknowledgements

Firstly, I'd like to thank my husband, Guy, for always supporting me in my creative work and being my own personal cheerleader. You're amazing and I love you.

I owe a special thanks to my beautiful friend Sammy, who first introduced me to this detox plan and showed me just how easy it could be to lead a healthy lifestyle and feel good from the inside out. #Healthywealthy

I'd love to thank the amazing people who shared their stories about how this detox plan has worked for them. Their willingness to share and bare all is truly inspiring. Thank you.

I'd also love to thank Ashley Pittman, Arbonne Regional Manager, for supporting me in this endeavour and helping me when I needed it via late night Voxer messages. Thanks for being open to new ideas!

Lastly, I want to thank you, dear reader, for taking a chance on this book and for saying "yes", to a healthier way of life for you. For trusting in yourself and your own ability to take care of you. You're the reason I wrote this book — YOU are amazing and inspirational to us all.

Table of Contents

Table of Contents

Foreword

Detox Your Diet. I couldn't have said it better myself!

As a physician and weight loss specialist, the principles outlined in **Detox Your Diet** reflect those that I teach patients in my everyday practice.

Knowing that yo-yo dieting is not only ineffective but counterproductive, in that it hinders metabolism and can psychologically trigger binge eating, I counsel my patients against it.

Instead, I subscribe to eating natural foods and implementing regular physical activity as a way of life. The *'10 Detox Foods'* listed in the *Detox Your Diet plan* are in alignment with foods that I regularly recommend.

Increasingly, the scientific community is recognizing the significant role that intestinal bacteria plays on our overall health. In fact, studies suggest that intestinal bacteria can be linked to a multitude of medical conditions.

In response, the medical community is growing in its support and promotion of intestinal health.

Evidence points to a connection between the foods we eat and the quality of our intestinal bacterial composition. Common elements of today's processed, fast-food diets are believed to be contributors to poor gut health. It is suggested that poor gut health is linked to a compromised immune system and inflammatory states, obesity, and decreased energy to name just a few maladies.

So what's the solution?

The 28-Day *Detox Your Diet* Plan that Lise outlines in this book is a great way to address this problem because you abstain from foods that have been associated with poor gut health.

As a weight loss and wellness doctor, I love that *Detox Your Diet* is about detoxification and improving gut health rather than *dieting* per se. And I also love that Lise's plan is very doable in that it's only 28 days and comes with several delicious food plans.

There is a natural transition between the 28 Day plan and the maintenance phase, which Lise clearly details.

I wholeheartedly agree with her recommendation of moderation using the 80/20 rule.

A lifestyle of moderation is my mantra because it is healthy and doable for all.

Always check with your doctor before undergoing any dietary regimen. But, in the absence of any medical restrictions, I am positive that *Detox Your Diet* will enhance your health and add vitality to your life!

Shauna Collins, MD
Medical Weight Loss & Obesity Treatment Physician and Author of *No More Dieting!*
www.NoMoreDieting.com

Introduction

Have you ever woken up in the morning and felt bloated, yet you didn't eat anything "bad" the day before?

Have you ever eaten a meal and then noticed, half an hour later or so, that you feel sluggish and super full?

And what about uncontrollable farting? No, just me? Oi...

Hi, I'm Lise Cartwright, full-time author, creative coach, and previous dieter.

I say previous dieter because I no longer need or want to diet. In fact, I eat what I want, when I want, and it's all because of this amazing 28-day healthy eating and detox plan that was introduced to me in late 2016.

I've never thought of myself as being overweight, but I have always felt uncomfortable in my own skin. I felt like eating food was causing me more harm than good, because every time I ate, I would immediately feel sluggish, bloated, or just plain fat.

I exercise five times a week, and for years, this didn't seem to be making a difference in my weight loss goals. Sure, I wasn't putting any weight on, but I wasn't losing any either.

And this was plain frustrating!

Does this sound familiar to you at all? Can you relate?

Whatever your situation is, we're all guilty of trying fad diets in the hopes that by some miracle, the weight will actually stay off this time.

I don't know about you but none of these diets ever stopped me from bloating or feeling sluggish either.

In fact, it didn't seem to matter if I was eating healthy food or not, I still felt sluggish, bloated, and just plain ol' yuck.

Low energy? Check.

Feeling unlovable and unsexy? Check, check.

Starting to hate my body...Ding, ding, ding!

Things really started to come to a head for me when my husband and I decided we'd like to start trying for a baby soon. I remember feeling horrified at the prospect of getting pregnant, getting "fat," having the baby, and then NEVER losing the baby weight plus the weight I already had.

As you can see from my before photos below, I wasn't exactly big, but in my eyes, I was. My driving force to finally find a way to lose this weight once and for all, was so I didn't have to worry about the extra weight I'd gain during my pregnancy. Plus, I wanted to feel healthy and be healthy for this pregnancy, given that it will be my first and I'm older (I'm over 37).

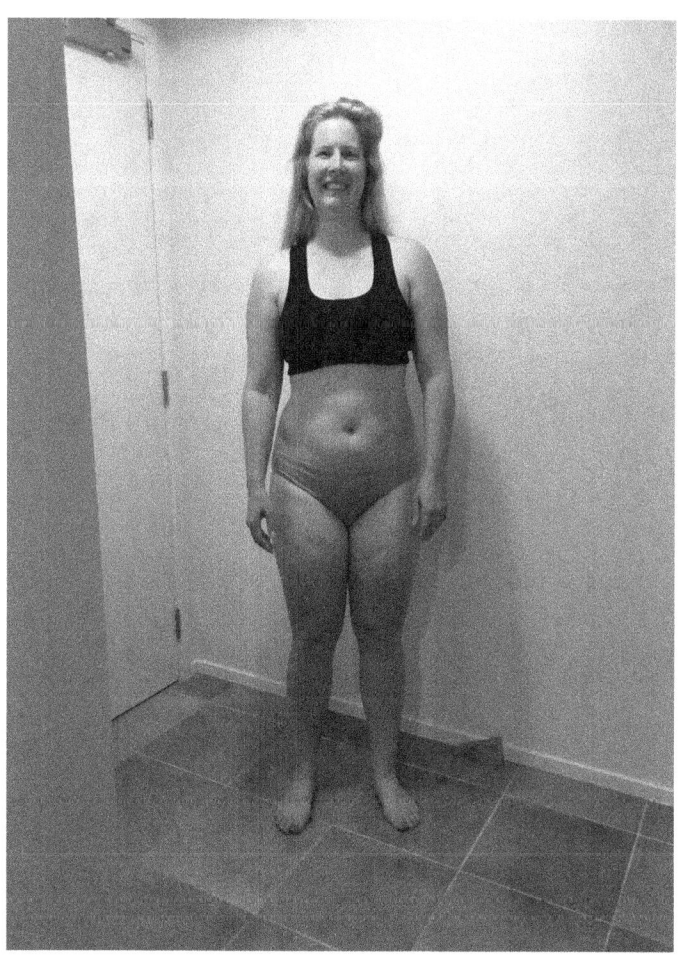

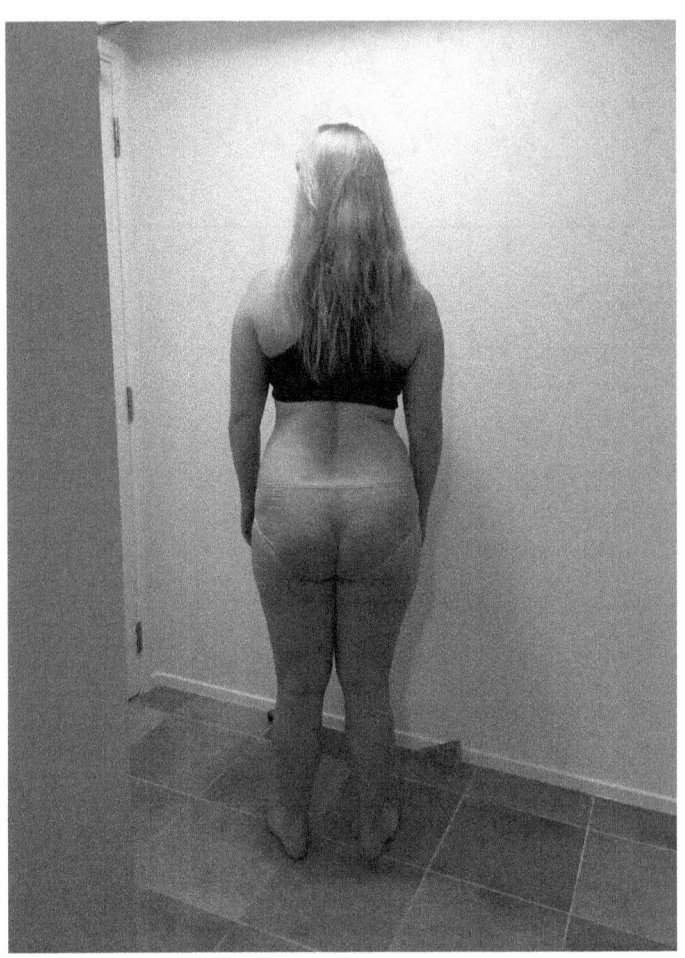

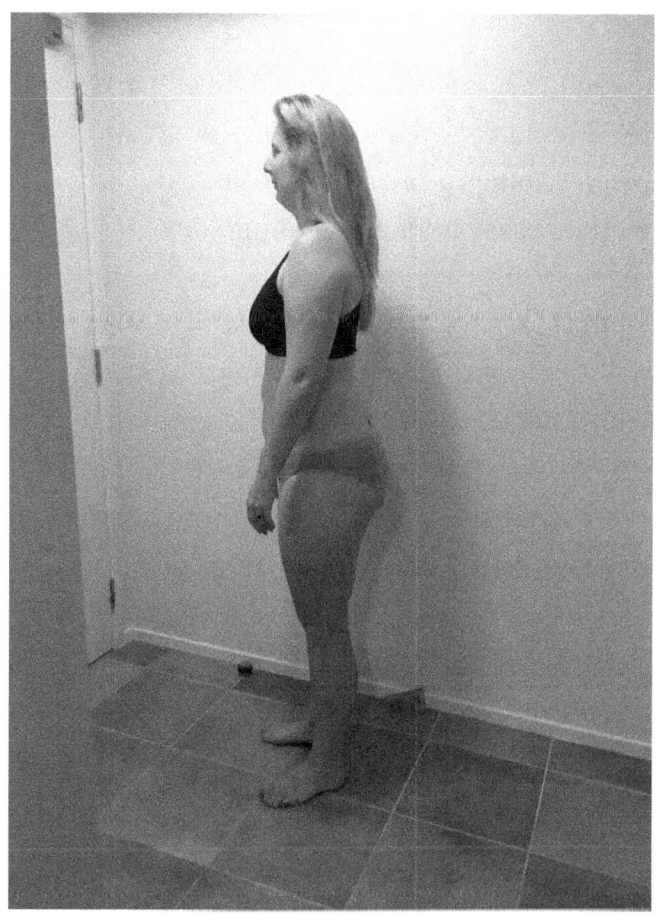

This time, when I started my research, I knew I wasn't looking for a diet. I was looking for a lifestyle change, a way to continue being healthy and maintaining an optimal weight, that didn't require buying foods I'd never heard of and spending hours in the kitchen.

Anyone that knows me well, knows how much I HATE to cook, so I was looking for solutions that weren't going to take a lot of time and would be relatively easy to implement into our lifestyle.

I gotta say, for a while I felt like there was NOTHING available that would work for me. Then I began to see a friend I'd met a few years ago through an educational program we took together, posting on Instagram the success she was having with this 28-day detox plan.

I was curious. My friend, Sammy, wasn't really carrying any extra weight, but she did experience some of the issues I did...bloating, feeling tired, having no energy, etc.

After chatting with her and doing my own research on the plan, I decided to give it a go...

What's outlined in this book is the EXACT plan Sammy shared with me. Since completing two 28-day detoxes, I've lost 10kgs (22 pounds), with more dropping as we speak!

I've lost 15 cms (six inches) around my hips, a similar amount around my waist... and in my thighs, where I tend to carry the most of my weight, I've lost 10 cms (four inches).

I FEEL amazing. I have so much energy, like my body clock has wound itself back to Lise, age 25. I'm keeping pace with 23-year-olds during my exercise classes, and people are commenting on how I look... how my skin is glowing and how healthy I look.

And those baby plans? They are back on the table again and we are getting in a lot of "practice" ;-)

Wondering how I'm looking now? Why don't you see for yourself...

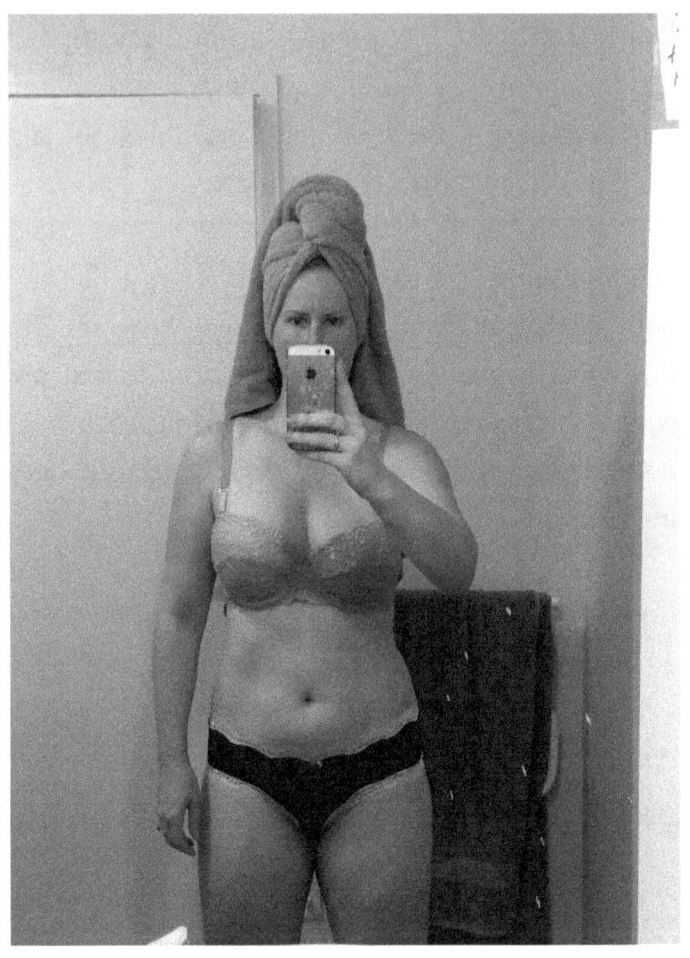

Why Dieting is Bad

Generally speaking, dieting is bad for us because of the following:

- Unsustainable long term
- Can make you gain even more weight
- Wreaks havoc with your digestive system
- Can be expensive to do

But don't take my word for it. Plenty of research has been conducted that shows why dieting is bad and why it doesn't even work.

For example, a study conducted in 1991 looked at the failure of behavioral and dietary treatments for obesity. It talks about the "overwhelming evidence that they are ineffective in producing lasting weight loss." [Source: ScienceDirect.com]

In a more recent study, UCLA professor Traci Mann led a meta study of 31 long term studies on dieters. She concluded that while most were able to lose weight (up to 10% of their starting body weight), within four to five years, they either regained all the weight lost, or gained even more. [Source: ScienceDaily.com]

Not only does dieting not even work, it's bad for your mental health too. If you're an ongoing dieter, you could be prone to elevated cortisol (stress hormone), which can lead to binge eating. [Source: US National Library of Medicine, National Institutes of Health]

I don't want to make this all doom and gloom, but I did want to point out how harmful dieting can be.

> *"There is no diet that will do what eating healthy does for your body."*

What you should be looking for are lifestyle changes — not a diet that will initially help you lose weight but doesn't provide you with sustainable lifestyle choices and changes for you to continue with AFTER you reach your optimal weight.

There's even a movement called The Anti-Diet Project, which you can check out at Refinery29: http://www.refinery29.com/the-anti-diet-project

We are all told to maintain a healthy diet...but what exactly does that even mean?

Thankfully, Google has the answer…

"A healthy diet contains a balance of food groups and all the nutrients necessary to promote good health." [Source: Wikipedia]

But what if you don't know what those are?! What then?

Well, don't worry. This book is going to teach you the skills you need to maintain a healthy diet without ever dieting again!

Why This Book?

Although this book is designed to help you lose

weight and adopt a healthier lifestyle, those goals require effort on your part. If you don't actually do the detox plan, nothing will change. It's as simple as that.

So stop right now and make a promise to YOURSELF that you'll stick with this for at least 14 days. Why 14 days? Because this will give you enough time to really feel the benefits and start to see changes.

Even if you've been exercising for a while or trying multiple diets at once, this book will still hit home for you in a way that other "diets" have not.

Here's what Lucy, a corporate executive from Dallas, Texas, had to say:

"After three days straight of traveling for work, I've lost weight. The detox plan makes it easy to stick to, even when I'm traveling. I ate at *Chipotle* for lunch, opting for the no-rice option. I couldn't be happier with how easy this is to implement."

The ideas and lifestyle changes suggested in this

book can be implemented and put into action by anyone, anywhere, and they will instantly provide you with ways to start feeling healthy TODAY.

Before you can really start your healthy lifestyle, you need to "detox your diet," which is what this book is all about.

Whether you're stuck working in an office, working from home, juggling multiple start-ups or jobs, or chasing the kids around the house, this detox and healthy lifestyle plan WILL work for you.

> *"Sooner or later, those who win are those who think they can."*
> *~ Richard Bach, bestselling author of Jonathan Livingston Seagull*

If you're sick of trying to figure this out on your own, sick of yo-yo and fad dieting, and feeling duped every time the weight returns, then you owe it to yourself to give the *Detox Your Diet* plan a go.

The reality is, you have nothing to lose and everything to gain.

I promise that if you follow the plan, stick to the "avoid" list and continue to exercise as you are now, you'll achieve your weight loss and health goals 3X faster than what you're currently doing.

You cannot fail if you follow the plan!

Not only that, but if you stick to the *Detox Your Diet* plan laid out in the book and implement the recipes and meal options (available in the free *Detox Friendly Action Guide*), you'll create new habits and see a change in how you approach your eating (and how you approach your food), leading to a healthier lifestyle and long term, sustainable weight loss.

Don't be the person who wishes they could change the way they look and feel, but doesn't do anything to make those necessary changes. Be the kind of person that inspires others to make healthier choices. Be the kind of person other

people see and say, "I don't know how they manage to look healthy and eat what they want!"

Be the kind of person who implements what they learn — who takes action and NEVER diets again.

You owe it to yourself and those you love.

The only people who shouldn't continue reading this book are those who already have the body and healthy lifestyle they want.

The *Detox Your Diet* plan you're about to learn about has been **proven to create body-changing and long-lasting results**.

All you have to do to achieve the same is to keep reading this book and take action.

Take back control of your body, your health, and your food right now. Make them work for you and create a body you love.

But don't take my word for it. Turn the page to read other people's success stories for more inspiration.

Testimonials & Success Stories

Before we get to the detox plan details, I'd love to share some success stories with you, from people who have gone through this exact process.

As mentioned, everyone's results will differ, but the key is that if you stick with the detox, you will see results.

Brad & Katie Benavides

I have been overweight since high school and I have always been active but it was never enough! Then I tried the 28-Day Detox Plan.

The shakes (using Arbonne's vegan protein) fill me up and the recipes are so easy to follow.

I have support every day through a private Facebook group, and am learning along the way why we shouldn't eat certain foods and what those foods are doing to our bodies.

With the 28-Day Detox Plan I lost 13 pounds and 2 1/2 inches on my waist, in 28 days.

I feel less bloated and have tons of energy, and since I just had a baby in August 2016 and also have a two-year-old to chase around, I need all the energy I can get!

I'm at month five now of following this healthy living plan and have lost a total of 30 pounds.

Also, getting rid of all the addictive foods made it easier to stay on track. I breastfeed, and Elaina rarely spits up food like when I used to eat bad food, and now that she's teething, I really think she has less swelling in her gums.

I'm off my blood pressure meds too.

My husband, Brad, has lost 22 pounds in his first 30 days and has now lost 50 pounds.

He had tons of injuries from high school sports and is now mostly joint pain free and has less swelling throughout his body and, rarely gets headaches and is less cranky too. 😜

Check out Katie's before and after photos

below.

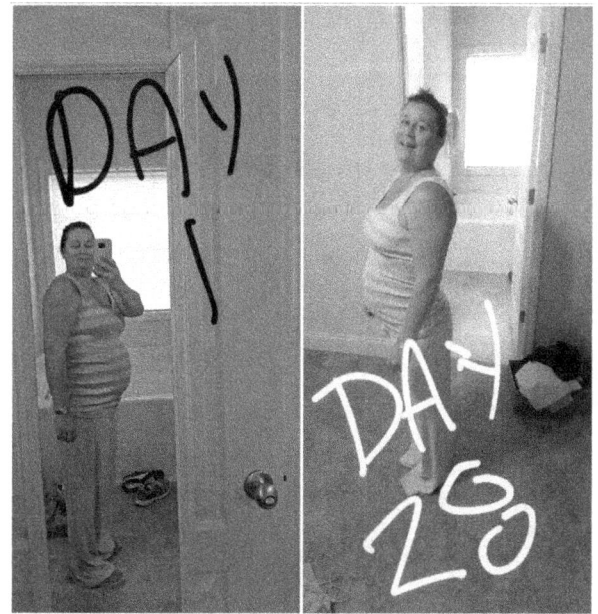

Katie's Before and After Pics

Rachel Gonzales

I started the 28-Day Detox Plan in February 2017.

I stepped off the scale this morning (March 16, 2017) and did waist measurements. I've lost 17 pounds and 5.5 inches off my belly.

Since starting the detox plan, my doctor has

pulled me off cholesterol and thyroid medication.

I have no more hot flashes/flushes, and my high blood pressure and migraines have disappeared...and that's just the start.

I'm absolutely in love with eating clean, and probably even more passionate and intense about the research, education, and resources [Arbonne] provides.

Never in a million years would I have believed 30 days would literally change my life.

My doctor told me at the end of January 2017, *"Stop running for your marathon training, because you will be the one dead at the finish line. Your cholesterol and pre-diabetic blood work is frightening and could be fatal if you keep doing what you are doing."* He wrote me five prescriptions and sent me on my way.

I was absolutely devastated, and then the following week, I was introduced to the 28-Day Detox Plan and vegan products...definitely divine intervention, wouldn't you agree?!

Check out Rachel's before and after photos below.

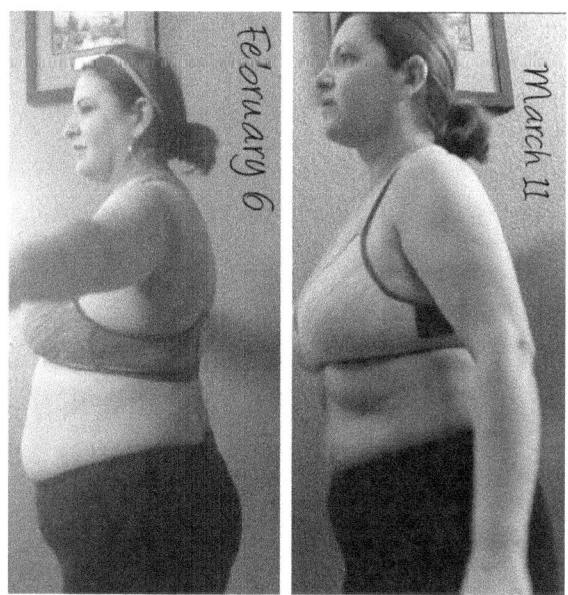

Rachel's Before & After Pics

Ed Miller

I've had some depression issues in my life and can sometimes be negative, so I was very interested in learning more about how a healthier diet might help.

Early last year (2016), I was diagnosed with prostate cancer. It was successfully treated and I am doing very well. Along with the prostate cancer, I found I have high blood pressure so I was put on blood pressure medication. I also have high cholesterol and take a medication for that in addition to another pill as a result of the prostate cancer. I also have issues with heartburn and acid reflux and take an over-the-counter drug for that.

In early December 2016, I started thinking about all the pills I am taking and my health issues. I thought, "If I continue to do nothing, what next?"

So I decided to give up drinking, which I did for 67 days, and I wanted to try to start eating a little healthier to try to loose some weight as well.

I also drank a lot of diet coke, which also is not good. I was putting a lot of garbage in my body.

I work in an office job and it was not

uncommon for me to go pick up some fast food for lunch. I did start packing healthy lunches, and without drinking, I was able to lose about 10 pounds very quickly.

However, I couldn't lose any more following the same routine, and in fact, gained a few pounds back. I just could not take off any more weight!

It was explained to me that I need to get the toxins out of my body in order to take off additional weight.

In February 2017, I began the 28-Day Detox Plan. I was super excited to get going!

I shared all the weekly meal plans and recipes with my wife, who was willing to cook the clean eating recipes.

My wife, Linda, was not fully on board with the plan, as she would not give up certain things, and also didn't take any of the recommended vegan nutrition supplements. However, she had no issues cooking and eating the food.

Early on, the hardest part for me was giving up my coffee. However, I quickly found out how the [Arbonne] fizz sticks and herbal detox tea gave me energy I needed, and within a few days, I didn't miss the coffee as much as I thought I would.

Also, as I stated, I used to drink a lot of diet coke and not enough water. During the detox I was told I should be drinking more water, so I like to have a little flavor in it to make it more drinkable. I put some lemon wedges in my water, and lemon is reportedly a good cleanse for your liver.

I started doing that and now am into drinking more water. I have no intention of going back to diet coke.

Another bad habit I had was to hit a vending machine for a snack. Now one of the other things I do is buy raw almonds and cashews for a snack instead. I also make sure I pack a good, healthy lunch with either left overs from our clean eating meal the night before or some veggies and fruit.

For breakfast, I've either been having a smoothie or shake with the [Arbonne] vegan protein powders, green powder, and fiber.

The best thing I have liked about the detox plan is you don't have to go hungry and you don't have to count calories or really keep track of anything if you don't want to.

The key is you have to learn what is good to put into your body and what you should not.

I've learned so much over the last month and really plan to keep on with the clean eating the majority of the time. I also plan to keep using the vegan protein and green powders.

When I started the plan I weighed 207 pounds and in four weeks have dropped 11 pounds and am down to 196 pounds.

I also had a 44" waste and am now down to 41.5". I actually had to buy some new jeans the other day as my jeans were getting to loose fitting. I went from a size 36 waist to a 34!!! All in one month!

I am super happy with my results and am going to keep going strong. My goal weight is 180 pounds, so I am going to keep working at it until I achieve it.

Remember how I said I had heartburn and acid reflux, well during the detox plan, it didn't bother me at all.

Instead of taking my medication for that every day, I cut it down to every other day.

One of my other goals is to try and get off some of my medication, or at a minimum, reduced dosages. I won't do that without my doctor's advice though. My next appointment is early May 2017 and I will discuss with her after results of blood tests, exam, etc.

But I'm confident that we'll be able to at least reduce the medication I'm on.

Check out Ed's before and after photos below!

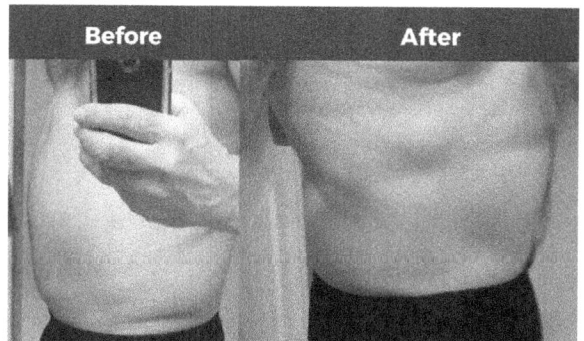

Ed's Before & After Pics

Simonne Tait

In 2014 I felt like I was living in a body that wasn't my own.

I was having a tough time moving, my head was constantly in a fog and I had ongoing digestion issues. I distinctly remember having to cancel plans to attend one of my best friends birthday dinners because I was so bloated that my joints hurt.

I was an otherwise healthy 32-year-old woman with no prior health issues. But I knew something was wrong, and if I didn't figure it out fast, I was for certain going to pop another button.

While sitting in the doctors office, in my stretchiest of stretch pants, I promised the weight loss gods that if I got a clean bill of health, I would put down the inflammation inducing foods and replace them with healthy food choices.

Unfortunately, I did not get a clean bill of health. The blood tests came back conclusive that my bad cholesterol (LDL) was off the charts, I was vitamin B and D deficient and the most devastating news was that I had moved from pre-diabetic to officially being diagnosed with Type 2 diabetes.

Needless to say, the scale tipped a few more pounds — several more pounds — than I expected.

I was shocked and ashamed, but more than anything, I was afraid.

Just a few weeks prior, I had lunch with my dear friend, Ashley Castle, Regional Vice President for

Arbonne. She introduced me to a healthy living 28-day challenge. I was excited to join the group and decided to take the step forward toward a cleaner and healthier lifestyle.

I shared with my doctor that I was starting a 28-Day wellness journey and she approved. We made an appointment to come back 30 days later and take the tests again to determine next steps.

The very next day I started my journey. I instantly fell in love with the [Arbonne] protein shakes. They were delicious and convenient for my on-the-go lifestyle. The fizz sticks were a life saver! I thought I would die without my 3:00pm coffee but the fizz sticks gave me a healthy energy boost without the crash from caffeine.

I started to feel my bloat dispel and was having the most restful nights. The first week was the most challenging, but by week two, I felt more like myself, even better!

On the final day of my detox journey I grabbed my chocolate protein shake and headed to my doctor. I hadn't stepped on a scale since I started the program, but I felt pretty confident sitting there in the waiting room that I wasn't going to pop any buttons!

My test results came back with very different results. My bad cholesterol was too low! I was no longer vitamin deficient and the biggest and best surprise of all — my blood sugar levels had dropped so much that I was no longer diabetic. I lost 27 inches all over and 13 pounds.

The 28-Day Detox and Arbonne's nutritional products gave me the gift of living a healthy lifestyle.

It was just the beginning of my journey though. I have since lost 50 pounds!

Motivation

Let's get real for a second. Eating healthy, living a better lifestyle, making changes in your life, these aren't easy.

Change is never easy. Is it worth it? Well, that really depends on you and WHY you're choosing to make a change.

Your motivation for doing a detox is what will keep you motivated throughout the next 28 days.

Because I'm not going to lie, the first week is hell, particularly if you've been eating a diet that mainly consists of all the "foods to avoid."

I get it. The first time I did this 28-day detox plan, I struggled with giving up sugar and gluten — like, S.T.R.U.G.G.L.E.D.

Sugar and me, we had this amazing relationship. All those tough times in my life when I was feeling horrible, or feeling lonely, or getting through a breakup… sugar was there to make me feel better.

All those happy times, birthday parties, Christmas, Easter...sugar was there to help me celebrate.

Sugar and I were joined at the hip — until I learned exactly what sugar was doing to my body.

I began to look at sugar with completely new eyes. It was like I'd been wearing dark glasses for the past 35 years and couldn't really see sugar for what it was...dangerous to my health.

I'll talk more about this (and the other foods to avoid) later on in the book, but just understand that motivating yourself to make this change isn't easy, but the results are so worth it.

As you already know, my main motivation for getting healthy is because we are looking to start a family, and as I'm a lot older than most first-time mothers, I know there is a higher risk.

I want to remove as many risks as possible by

making sure I'm in my most optimal, healthiest form, so that when I do fall pregnant, I know I've done everything I can to create a healthy environment for a great pregnancy.

This motivation, this understanding, is what kept me on track.

Did I crave sugar and all those "yummy" foods? Heck yes. I craved them so bad, but I also knew I could do without them for the next 28 days, and if at the end of this time I wanted to eat them again, I could.

Your motivation will be different.

If you truly want to make a change, you will. Your mind is strong. Your will is strong. You are strong.

YOU CAN DO THIS.

But, if you need extra help and strategies, I've brought in some other experts to share their wisdom too.

Read on to find out more.

Inspiration and Strategies

Words of Wisdom From Michelle Joy

Some great ways to stay motivated are to find other people on the same journey as you. It can be by recruiting a friend to join you in being healthier, or getting in touch with people online who are going through a similar process as you.

The aim is to find someone to keep you accountable and who can relate with you about the ups and downs of the journey.

For some people it helps to find that dream outfit or bathing suit they want to wear when they've hit their goals. For others it might be a certain amount of weight they'd like to lose, or sometimes just a number on the scale.

However, I would suggest you go more for a look and feel than just a number. Taking measurements and progress pictures are one of the most motivating things for me.

Being able to see the changes and look back and truly be amazed by what you've accomplished is so satisfying.

Vision/dream boards are also a great motivator.

Maybe you've got that cruise coming up or your high school reunion or you want to look spectacular for some certain event.

There are countless visual aids on Pinterest. One idea is to have a jar of pebbles, which you move from the "pounds to lose" to the "pounds lost" jar. This allows you to visually see your own process.

I can't stress enough how helpful it is to have accountability partners. Someone who will give you that nudge when you're feeling lazy, or who has been there with you every step of the way and can truly appreciate how much you have gone through to get to that victory, on the scale or off.

Reward systems are also useful. Maybe when

you hit a certain goal or do a particular number of workouts you get to buy those new workout shorts you really like, or a new pair of running shoes.

Find your WHY.

Do you want to make sure you can run and play with your kids? Or maybe you want to make sure you're healthy enough that you live to see them grow up and have kids of their own.

Maybe you want to feel like you can do anything you need to physically do and not be unable to care for yourself.

Work hard and then show off that body you busted your butt for. Find something that drives you and put that on the wall or on your mirror. See it every day so you keep pushing yourself to get closer every day.

Set goals like "lose three inches off my waist" or "run 10 minutes without stopping," and then set mini goals you can hit so that you keep the motivation going.

If you only have one final end goal, it can be hard to stay motivated. But if you have smaller goals, you can hit them and get excited again.

Do whatever it takes to be the healthier and happier you that you want to be. Get rid of the temptations, switch bad habits out for healthier ones. And never give up.

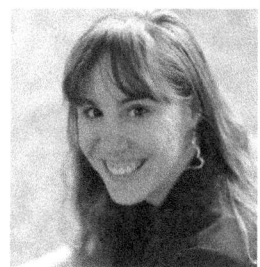

I'm Michelle Joy and I am an Independent Beachbody Coach. I workout and motivate people online and in person through their health and fitness journeys.

Connect with Michelle here:
- www.facebook.com/coachmichellejoy
- www.beachbodycoach.com/usfjoygirl

Strategies & Tips From Chalene Bezzina

All three strategies below are rather simple, but within that lies the beauty of it. We are busy people with busy lives and as such, find it hard to stick to things.

When we simplify tasks we are more likely to stick to them. And it's sometimes in doing the simplest of things that we learn the most.

#1: Track things

I love mentioning this to people as I am ironically one of those who's atrociously bad at doing it.

What I do know, though, is how much more successful and motivated I am throughout the process of attaining my goal if I track certain aspects of it.

It keeps me focused and clear on where I am at, and it's a great reminder to do little things toward your goals each day.

I personally use all the strategies suggested

below, which I've found negates the feelings of negativity associated with this particular task.

Tracking weight loss, water consumption, and/or calorie intake can be a little ho-hum. But getting a little more creative with things can do wonders for staying interested and continuing on with your journey.

A beautiful way to track things (for the right-brained folk) is by colouring in. You can do this by allocating days, weeks, or amounts to sections within your picture and then as you achieve them, you colour in a section.

This gives you a beautiful visual confirmation of your progress.

Something a little quicker and for the less creatively inclined, could be keeping a simple daily or weekly tally of your successes. This can be done in a monthly, weekly, or daily journal where you just jot down your progress as you go.

If you'd rather use a spreadsheet with crisp black

writing on a white background to tickle your fancy, then by all means go for it!

Doing this in a specially allocated diary or journal can be very beneficial; you're setting aside an area both physically and mentally for your goal.

Both methods are also great for future reference should you ever doubt your abilities to stick with things. It just takes looking back at your past progress to get you out of a motivational slump.

#2: Remind yourself why you're doing this

It seems like something very simple to do, but this can be a great sticking point for many.

We are very good at creating the illusion that the gratification we so desperately seek will last for longer than it will.

Upon reminding ourselves why we have chosen to make the changes we are wanting, we not only get ourselves out of a "craving funk," but perhaps tap into something a little deeper that may have triggered the craving in the first place.

Did someone say something to annoy you and you are now seeking to skip a planned meal? Or are you down due to something that happened during the day, causing your motivation for exercise to slump?

Always ask yourself why you are seeking the instant gratification (as you're reaching for that cookie) and listen to the answers that pop up.

On a surface level, it is great to stay motivated. On a sub level you may just uncover a gem that will allow you to dig deeper and understand yourself a little better.

By practicing delayed gratification (i.e., sticking with our goal — not eating the cookie), we create longer term rewards in the future (i.e., we succeed at attaining our goal — weight loss, healthier habits, fitter, etc).

Staying motivated is a funny thing. It is one of those subjects that there has been much discussion on, and what keeps each of us motivated varies from person to person.

Within this falls a powerful question I read a while ago that has stuck with me ever since:*"Is this serving me right now?"*

What I love most about this simple question is twofold.

One, it reminds you that you are doing this for yourself; you have set a goal that serves YOU, and you're the one who's going to make or break it.

Second, it is a quick yet effective way for you to bring focus back to the "why" of the situation, whatever it may be. And it's rather easy too.

All you have to do is put the sentence where it can be seen every day. When you want to sleep in but know you have to get up for yoga, glance at the question... *"Is this serving me right now?"*

When you're eyeballing that sugary treat that you know you shouldn't have, glance at the question... *"Is this going to serve me right now?"*

In all instances, the question brings you back to thinking about actions and consequences.

Are you honouring yourself and sticking to your journey to create change? Are you honouring your "why" for initially starting this goal?

This isn't an activity meant to guilt trip you into obedience, but rather as a quick reminder to keep you on track.

#3: Be gentle on yourself

This to me is of the utmost importance.

Living in the twenty-first century has allowed women to start rising up and owning their own feminine power in what is still a predominantly masculine world.

Similarly, men in today's world are dealing with the increasing acceptance of males being more emotionally expressive. (I say "deal" as it can be a little overwhelming coping with your own or others' repressed emotions when they are finally allowed to surface.)

With this comes its own set of challenges. I think it is safe to say that whether you believe in the spiritual world or not, you've noticed that change is in the air.

We want to do things our own way, but the majority of us still have a very patriarchal approach to actioning things. This approach isn't wrong, but with it can come a sense of personal lack, a sense of disempowerment, and feelings of "not enough"; particularly if we feel we are failing.

As women or men in the twenty-first century, we are learning that things can still get done, and sometimes a whole lot more efficiently, if we are more gentle on ourselves.

The act of being gentle with oneself can differ between men and women, but underpinning it all is allowing flow to come into your life.

The endless push to get things done is not always needed. Having a break, taking five, doing something that is FUN and SIMPLE can sometimes be the better approach.

Or quite literally, just *going with the flow*.

It needs to be done without a sense of guilt or worry. We all want to achieve our goals and make our dreams come true, but we need balance.

Within this balance we have to honour ourselves by stepping back and having a breather without the guilt and worry that we aren't doing enough.

We all need rest. We all need relaxation. We all need fun. Make sure to add these into your goal "game plan" too.

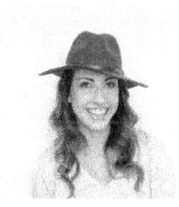 As a life coach Chalene focuses on women struggling with change to succeed in realizing their potential, and help them get their inner power, confidence and strength back.

Connect with Chalene here:

- http://www.instagram.com/nelizak

- http://www.neliza-k.com

Illuminating and Inspiring Ideas From Marsha Lodge

We are aware that maintaining a healthy lifestyle requires concentration and commitment. It takes time to build up this sort of trust and confidence, so please do not expect any overnight miracles.

If your goal is weight loss, please bear in mind that you did not gain the weight overnight so you must be patient with yourself when trying to lose it. Go easy on yourself. It takes self-discipline and a reconditioning of the mind to accomplish positive results.

You have to unlearn and develop a new way of living and this requires time, patience, and a positive attitude.

The ideas below are strategies that have helped me in my own wellness journey.

Why

One of the first steps in staying motivated with

this program or any other, for that matter, is to know and affirm your whys.

Why am I doing this detox?

Speak your reasons why out loud so you can hear them and write them down so you can remember them.

Your whys are very important; once you have established them the how will take form. There is no how without a why.

Whys are the driving forces to the how. And once you have distinguished your purpose, your actions will align and begin to manifest.

Honesty
Honesty to self is important. Confront yourself on the things that are stopping you: self-doubt, laziness, time. Whatever those things are, see them for exactly what they are: excuses.

You must understand and believe that within you is the power to do anything you set your mind to. You are limitless, and the only thing stopping you is you.

Acknowledge your current lifestyle and your attachments, especially your relationship with food.

Psychoanalyze and evaluate yourself authentically, allowing space for vulnerability and acceptance.

Take accountability for your role in your own life. And make an affirmed decision to begin your journey.

It's important that you know that change requires honesty and in order to change our bad habits, we must change our frequency. We must be honest.

Reconditioned Attitude and Mindset
With honesty comes a shift in attitude, an openness to change, to reset and recondition our thought process. This is reestablishing a new mindset geared more toward our intentions.

We begin to break down the barriers as we now

recognize what is standing between us and our goals.

With this program, you will become informed in ways that will only expand your awareness; awareness of self, health, diet, and mindset.

You will begin to change your language to one that aligns more with your intentions, a language that's geared more toward success, a language that inspires and motivates, a language of self love and discipline.

You will feel a shift happening within your way of being and ultimately your consciousness.

To stay on track with this plan, you must be willing to unlearn what you have believed as truth and reeducate yourself, acknowledging newfound facts and insights into what is the actual truth.

We have been fed a lot of false information (around the foods we eat) all or most of our lives, mostly for the benefit of capitalistic gains.

An acknowledgment of this fact doesn't mean you are a "conspiracy theorist." It means you are a realist, and you are now aware and will not buy into the lies any longer.

It means you will take affirmative action as it relates to your health. We have been vastly manipulated through commercialization, and until we begin to break the chains wrapped around our minds, we will never obtain and sustain good health.

Mindfulness
Mindfulness is a state of being mindful or aware. Psychologically, it's a technique in which one focuses one's full attention only on the present.

Let's apply mindfulness to our eating habits. Apply it to this plan.

Consider yourself mindful when you sit down to create your grocery list, when you go to the grocery store to shop, when you step into the kitchen to prepare your meal, and when you sit down to eat.

Consider yourself present, aware, and knowledgeable.

This is how you create the space for mindful eating. We have control, and we become aware of this fact through information and mindfulness.

We begin to understand the effect a certain food has on our bodies, whether negatively or positively, and we begin to adjust our actions accordingly.

Because the mind has shifted into a more elevated state of consciousness, we begin the work.

We do not just point fingers at large food corporations and pharmaceutical companies; we begin to hold ourselves accountable as well.

We begin to understand that our health is our responsibility and the only true wealth we possess. It opens us up to DOING.

Mindfulness creates balance and balance is essential in all that we do. It sustains the operation and continuation of life.

We have to create balance and awareness within ourselves for it to manifest in our actions. What we think, do, and speak affects everything in our life. Your diet is part of that frequency.

The things we put into our bodies highly affect other aspects of our human existence. Those things can weaken the mind, the body, and the spirit, respectively. So we must become mindful that our diet aids in creating balance in our life.

It is connected to our consciousness.

This program proposes a way for you to CHANGE YOUR DIET. A way to access information and become more knowledgeable and experienced in taking care of our nutritional health.

It offers a way to become more aware and committed to a complete lifestyle change. This isn't just about 28 days out of your life. This is about the rest of your life.

"Selfullness" is a word I created because, to be

successful on this journey or anything else, you have to be committed to yourself, to your well-being. You will need to be stronger than your desire.

Napoleon Hill says, *"The starting point of all achievement is desire."*

Selfullness starts in the mind; conditioning your mind to do whatever it takes to fully experience the life you desire. If you can conquer your mind, you can do absolutely anything you set out to do.

This program will help you tap into that frequency so that once the 28 days have passed, you will never go back to old bad habits.

You will experience a rebirth. You must exercise self-discipline, and you must acquire the knowledge and infuse that knowing into your everyday life.

You must be accountable for yourself. This is about YOU, so really, the most essential requirement here is YOU. You must become mindful of yourself.

Self Love

Love begins from within and then transcends. Believe you are worthy of good health and capable of achieving and sustaining it.

Loving yourself enough to do what's best for you is a source of divine power. It will get you through absolutely anything.

The power of self love can transform your entire life. It's like an evolution of attitude and perception. You will begin to see your magic and claim your worthiness.

Self love is a practice. It's a method of breaking old patterns that no longer serve you and creating new ideas and dimensions of yourself.

It is the power of believing in yourself, knowing you have what it takes to get it done. Knowing you deserve the rewards and benefits that come with getting it done.

Self love is one of the most powerful and effective tools needed to stay in commitment, with this or any other challenges we face in life. You get to affirm yourself every day.

It's being responsible for life, your intentions, your actions, and your results; loving yourself is easy when you've accepted yourself. Loving yourself is natural because you are the one person you cannot live without.

We all possess the power to heal ourselves and transform ourselves into happy, healthy, purposeful human beings. The time to live well is now. Are you ready to recondition your lifestyle?

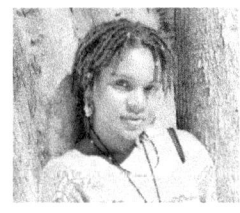

Marsha is an Arbonne Consultant and Wellness Coach. Having lupus has helped open her consciousness to the fact that we have an obligation to help one another to create a lifestyle of mindfulness, health, and wellness.

Connect with Marsha here:

- http://wellnessrebirth.ontrapages.com/livingwellnow
- https://www.instagram.com/wellnessrebirth/

Why "Detox Your Diet?"

It's highly likely that you've picked up this book because you want to lose weight or want to be healthier...but I also bet underlying that is the want (need?) to feel good from the inside out.

Our bodies are pretty amazing. They are custom-built to keep us running in optimal condition... *provided* we fuel up on the right foods.

And therein lies the problem.

But it's not necessarily all our fault either. After all, how often have you had good intentions of buying something healthy, only to get to the supermarket and find that the healthier option is super expensive?

You end up buying the unhealthier option because it's a budget thing. And no-one can blame you for that; I've done it too.

Or maybe you're not even sure what is healthy and what isn't. There are a lot of grey areas when it comes to packaging information and in some cases, unless you're a scientist, you have NO IDEA what's in the food you're eating.

Which is why you need to educate yourself. Remember how I said it wasn't all our fault? This is true to the extent that most of us can't read or understand the scientific words that are listed on most food labels...but we do still have to take responsibility for what we put in our bodies.

We can educate ourselves on packet labels and find out what those listed ingredients actually mean.

If you want your body to detox itself properly, then you need to feed it the right food.

Dr. Alejandro Junger, MD, says, "The first thing a good detox does is corrects intestinal health."

Without good intestinal health, a.k.a. a good digestive system, your body's detox process isn't able to work properly. Instead, what happens?

Bad bacteria. It starts to stay in our bodies when we can't eliminate it. And the worst part? Some

of the foods we're eating on a daily basis are feeding the bad bacteria!

This bad bacteria leads to fat storage and absorption and also causes our bodies to be more acidic.

> *"Every single person who has cancer has a pH that is too acidic."*
> *~ Dr. Otto Warburg, Nobel Prize Winner, 1931*

This is why a lot of diets don't work — because your digestive system isn't able to deal with good foods due to all the bad bacteria that's built up from years of eating "bad" foods.

This makes so much sense to me. It explains why, in my younger years, I would eat things like breads and pastas and not gain weight...but as I got older, weight began to stick around and get harder to move.

By the time I was 35, I was 15kgs (33 lbs)

heavier than I was at age 16, and I felt extremely sluggish. Yet I couldn't put my finger on why. Sure, I would eat crap food here and there, but for the most part, I was eating what I thought were healthy foods...

I also spent a lot of time exercising and still wondered why nothing was changing. I wasn't gaining any weight, but I certainly wasn't losing it either.

Since I implemented the *Detox Your Diet* plan, I've been able to lose weight, feel energized, and have a body I truly adore. I've also noticed a shift in the way I look at food and the way food tastes. Will the same happen for you? Probably, but results will vary as everyone is different.

What I can tell you is that, without doing a detox like this first, there is no way that you'll be able to lose and keep weight off long term.

Benefits of Detoxing

A good detox plan creates conditions for your organs and intestinal systems to detox effectively and optimally.

Once you've gone through the detox phase, you can then begin to focus on weight loss and eating cleaner foods.

Below are some of the "side effects" of following this 28-Day Detox Plan:

#1: Weight Loss

Weight loss is obviously the biggest benefit of detoxing, but if you don't review your lifestyle and change the way you eat, the detox will be ineffective, because as soon as you start eating foods that feed bad bacteria, the faster you'll start to put weight back on.

So you need to review both your eating and your lifestyle in conjunction with this detox plan to ensure you achieve healthy weight loss...forever.

#2: Correct Digestive System

In order to stay healthy and get rid of bad bacteria, we need our digestive system to function properly. If you currently suffer from bloating or certain foods upset your tummy, then a detox and clean eating plan is going to make you feel like a new person from the inside out.

Without your digestive system working properly, losing weight is difficult.

And while I've never been diagnosed with Irritable Bowel Syndrome (although apparently it is sensitive!), I do suffer from bloating and a very irregular bowel. Too much information?!

While it might seem that way, I believe it's important that you understand exactly where I started from when I did this detox plan so that you can decide for yourself if it's the right option for you.

It was and is, without a doubt, the right option for me. And I KNOW it will be for you.

#3: Regulate Menstrual Cycle

Sorry to all the men reading this book, but this has to be addressed! You can skip to the next point.

TMI alert! I've been on the contraceptive pill since I was 13. The reason I went on it wasn't because I was sexually active, but because I had my period for an entire 30 days, during summer, and I had had enough of it...so had my mother!

I also suffered from extreme abdominal cramps, having to stay home from school in the first few days of my period.

While this lessened as I got older, the abdominal cramps could sometimes come in very sharp, breath-taking bursts...but as any of you ladies can attest, you learn to live with it.

When I started the detox plan, I'd literally just finished my period. Within seven days of being on the detox plan, I got my period again!

You can imagine how that went down, lol. I wasn't impressed. But I quickly learned from my nutritionist that this type of detox plan not only detoxes your digestive system, but ALL your systems.

So while I'd just had my period, this one I was experiencing now was part of the detox process and not a "real" period.

After it finished about seven days later, I didn't give it a second thought...until my next period arrived, like clockwork, 21 days later. The most amazing part about this?

NO PERIOD PAIN! For the first time in 26 years, I was experiencing no abdominal cramping, no tender breasts, and no sharp pains.

In fact, I was quite surprised when my period arrived, because I hadn't been expecting it. I had used the abdominal cramps and tender breasts as signs that it was on its way.

Not any more! Now I'm a "normal" gal who can monitor her cycle and not worry about the crappy bits.

I'd like to point out that I'm not a doctor, so if you're at all worried about something like this happening, please seek medical advice first.

Menopausal? Then you may find yourself having your own "not really a period" period too.

The detox will help regulate things for you and should help with all those annoying symptoms like hot flushes/flashes and hormonal imbalances. But remember, results vary from person to person.

The important thing is to record EVERYTHING while on the detox, but we'll chat more about that later.

#4: Regulate Body's Detox System

A good detox plan supports the body's own systems. Our bodies generate and retain fat to protect us, and detoxing helps to get rid of bad fats while keeping the good.

Without the ability to detox, our bodies store bad fats, which feed the bad bacteria hanging around in our tummies… It's a vicious cycle.

My nutritionist recommends doing a detox two-three times a year to make sure your system is working optimally.

The *Detox Your Diet* Philosophy

Before we jump into the nitty gritty details of the detox plan, I want to highlight the philosophy behind this plan.

First things first, this isn't about starving yourself! This detox plan is about supporting your digestive system and teaching you how to eat cleanly. No calorie counting here.

This is also, as I've already mentioned during the introduction, not a fad or crash diet. They are bad for your system and will only provide short term weight loss results.

We're looking for long term results here people, am I right?!

The main philosophy behind this detox plan is eliminating the foods that are not good for you, the foods that feed bad bacteria. These tend to be foods that cause acidity in the body and are unnatural, i.e., not foods we would be able to access if we were living in the wild.

Once we eliminate those foods, we then replace

them with clean foods, foods that encourage good bacteria to flourish and support our organs and internal systems in operating at optimal levels.

Allowing our bodies to regulate our own detox systems.

We do this for 28 days to allow our bodies time to eliminate the bad bacteria and get back on track. If, like me, you've had years of eating the "bad'"foods, you might need to repeat this detox for a further 28 days.

Part of this plan does include nutritional products designed to support all your internal functions. They are optional, but will bring you the best and fastest results. You can learn more about these at www.detoxyourdietplan.com.

And lastly, before we get started, there is a level of exercise expected to help move your body as part of the detox process.

You don't have to do the exercises but you SHOULD incorporate some level of mild exercising while following the detox plan, if only to support your muscles and bones.

I mean, what's the point in getting your body's detox system working optimally if you're not going to take full advantage of all the extra energy you're going to have? Not too mention that if you want to live a long and happy life, you need your bones and muscles healthy too.

I know you're probably thinking, "Enough already, Lise! Let's get this party started!"

Ok then. Time to turn the page and dive right in!

Detox

Your Diet

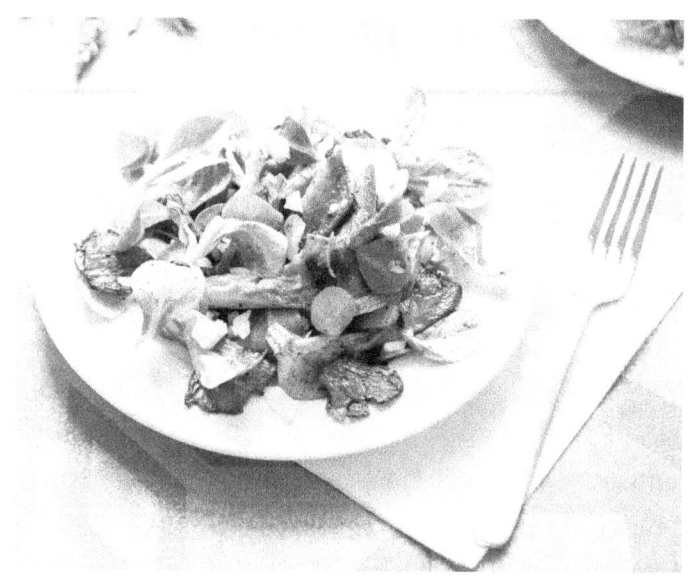

A 28-Day Detox Plan

Getting Started

When we are born, our bodies are brand new and working in optimal condition. Then, as we begin to grow, we start being introduced to different types of foods, and for most of us, that means bread, meat, vegetables, fruit, pasta, and sweets.

While we are fit, young, and healthy, everything is working great. We're able to maintain energy levels, think proactively, and "eat what we like" without any (noticeable) consequences.

But then, something happens — you notice a small shift at first, maybe in your late 20s, then you're about 35 and wondering how on earth you could be carrying an extra 15-20 kgs (33-44 lbs).

You've always had a pretty healthy diet, although you do like to indulge in the odd sweet here and there and come the weekend, you're letting loose and enjoying a few (ok, a lot) glasses of wine or beer.

them with clean foods, foods that encourage good bacteria to flourish and support our organs and internal systems in operating at optimal levels.

Allowing our bodies to regulate our own detox systems.

We do this for 28 days to allow our bodies time to eliminate the bad bacteria and get back on track. If, like me, you've had years of eating the "bad"'foods, you might need to repeat this detox for a further 28 days.

Part of this plan does include nutritional products designed to support all your internal functions. They are optional, but will bring you the best and fastest results. You can learn more about these at www.detoxyourdietplan.com.

And lastly, before we get started, there is a level of exercise expected to help move your body as part of the detox process.

You don't have to do the exercises but you SHOULD incorporate some level of mild exercising while following the detox plan, if only to support your muscles and bones.

I mean, what's the point in getting your body's detox system working optimally if you're not going to take full advantage of all the extra energy you're going to have? Not too mention that if you want to live a long and happy life, you need your bones and muscles healthy too.

I know you're probably thinking, "Enough already, Lise! Let's get this party started!"

Ok then. Time to turn the page and dive right in!

Nothing that would make you put on that much weight, surely?

Uh, I hate to tell you this, but if your body's detox system is overwhelmed with bad bacteria, it can't deal with it fast enough. And then you're adding more bad bacteria to it (through what you're eating), to the point where your body is barely able to properly digest and process the foods you're eating.

Is it any wonder we're carrying extra weight?!

If our bodies can't detox and process the foods we're eating, this leads to weight gain and longer term health issues. Bloating, constipation, gas, feeling sluggish, these are all symptoms of a detox system that is struggling.

This is why you're here.

To make healthy decisions, you need to have knowledge about the foods you're eating, and a supportive digestive system to help process those foods.

Before you can lose weight, you need to get your body's detox system up and running properly, which means for the next 28 days, things are going to be tough.

But if you want to feel good, have more energy and vitality, lose weight, and live a long and happy life, 28 days is nothing in comparison with what you'll gain.

So with that in mind, let's jump into the 'meat and potatoes' of the Detox Your Diet plan.

The Basics

To start with, we're going to eliminate foods that cause bad bacteria in your system. These foods either increase the acidity of your body (which helps grow bad bacteria) or they feed the bad bacteria.

Think of bad bacteria as little gremlins inside

your digestive system and elimination organs, gorging on the following foods that they love to eat and that suck your energy because your body's detox system is working in overdrive to get rid of them!

Step 1: Eliminate "bad" foods

- dairy/eggs
- gluten/wheat
- processed sugar
- soy
- coffee/soda/alcohol
- beef/pork
- corn
- peanuts

The aim is to go cold turkey on these foods. Remove them all at the same time. The first few days will be tough, but then things will get easier, I promise.

The main reason these foods are removed from our diets is because they cause acidity in the body and feed bad bacteria in our gut.

We put weight on when we have too much of the

bad bacteria built up in our system. If you eat the toxic foods above on a regular basis, you are feeding the bad bacteria and clogging up your detox system.

By removing the toxic food mentioned above, you stop feeding the bad bacteria and allow good bacteria to grow and flourish in its place.

And that's a good thing, because when we have more good bacteria than bad, our body's detox system kicks in and helps us get rid of excess fat and toxins by eliminating them from your body.

Don't fight me on this step!

These foods are like poison to your body. The more you eat of them, the more weight you'll gain.

If you want more energy and to lose weight, stick to this plan and eliminate these foods...at least for the next 28 days.

You at least owe it to yourself to try.

Step 2: Replace with good foods

Now that we've eliminated those foods, you're probably wondering what you can eat!

Below are the foods you should consume throughout the next 28 days.

10 Detox Foods

1. green leafy vegetables (these are the king of the detox foods)
2. cold water fish
3. free range chicken
4. berries (fresh or frozen)
5. apple cider vinegar/green apples (helps digestion)
6. lemon water (helps increase alkaline levels in your body)
7. herbal teas (boosts energy)
8. coconut milk/almond milk
9. coconut oil/olive oil
10. plant-based (pea/rice) protein powder (helps your liver work effectively)

And we're not counting calories here either! Instead, stick to filling your plate as follows:

- 50% veggies (like kale, spinach, broccoli, asparagus)
- 25% lean protein (like legumes, lentils, free-range chicken, cold water fish, or turkey)
- 12.5% complex carbs (like brown rice, quinoa, beets, sweet potatoes, carrots, or millet)
- 12.5% good fats (like seeds, nuts, nut butters, nut oils, olive oil, avocado, flax, grape seed oil, coconut oil)

See the image opposite for a visual reference point.

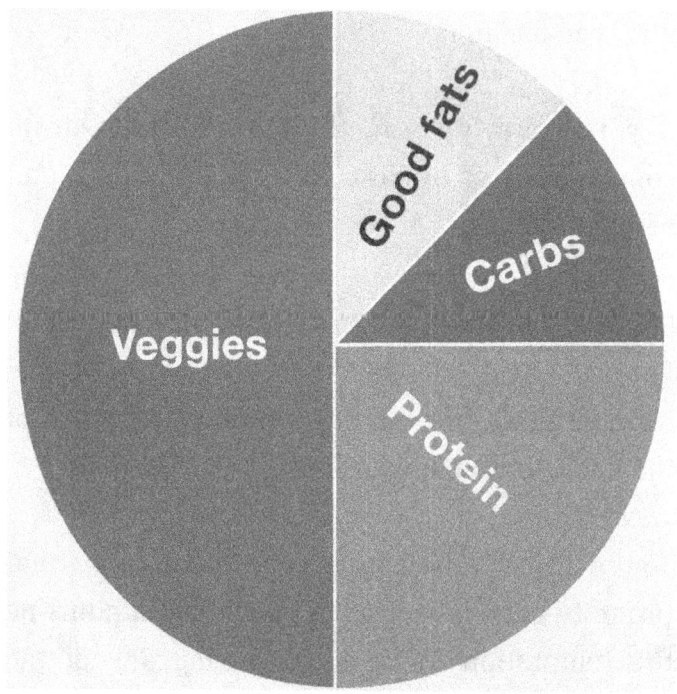

By eating these foods throughout the next 28 days, the workload is reduced on your digestive system, which means it can work on getting rid of the bad bacteria in your body.

This is what will help you to feel great and lose weight.

Step 3: Eat until you're full

Remember, we're not counting calories during this 28-day detox plan. The aim is simply to eat until you feel full.

If you're craving something sweet, then drink some herbal tea or eat a good fat, like a teaspoon of almond butter.

Step 4: Cleanse the elimination organs

For the first two weeks, you're going to be training your body to start eliminating more of the bad bacteria in your body.

You're going to be eating good, clean foods that promote good bacteria, and you'll be minimizing the temptation to revert to eating any of the eliminated foods.

At the beginning of week three, you're going to drink a special herbal tea to help you cleanse your liver properly.

You'll still be eating clean foods and drinking plenty of water, but in addition to this, you'll be drinking an herbal cleansing tea every day for seven days.

Step 5: Move that body

In the first week of the plan, you should aim to reduce or do minimal exercise. The reason for this is that your body will be working overtime to get rid of all the bad bacteria. If you spend your energy exercising, it will take longer for the body to get back to optimal detoxing.

So in the first week, light to no exercise only.

But in the following weeks, increase your exercise! Aim for at least 30 minutes of high intensity workouts, three to five times a week.

You can see some ideas for exercising in *Chapter Seven: Exercise Options*.

Now that we've covered the basics, below is some further information on what you can expect to happen to your body during the next 28 days...

What to Expect

I know you're super excited to get started, but as I've already alluded to, the detox plan can be tough to stick to, and not just because you're probably cutting out a lot of your favorite foods.

Initially, you might feel pretty crap. And while this might seem counterintuitive, it's a good thing, because it means your body is detoxing and the detox plan is kicking in.

In the first week, you could experience some of the following:

Severe headaches. This is generally due to sugar and caffeine withdrawals. Drink lots of water and push through it; you'll feel a lot better in two to three days.

Constipation and/or diarrhoea. This can happen as you increase the amount of fiber you're eating.

Make sure you're drinking at least half your bodyweight in water. This will help flush your system out and move fiber along the digestive track.

The aim is to have two to three bowel movements per day. This is a main process of your body's detox system, so this needs to be working well.

If symptoms haven't disappeared within two to three days, seek medical advice.

Strong body odor. Your body will sweat out toxins too, so if you're at the stage where you're increasing your exercise activities, you might notice that your sweat smells stronger.

Continue to drink more water or head to a sauna to help your organs of elimination process this faster.

Swollen lymph nodes. If you've got a lot of bad bacteria built up in your system, or too much yeast build up, then you may notice tender or swollen lymph nodes.

This means your immune system is joining the detox fight to rid your body of an infection. To help your lymph nodes eliminate these faster, try jumping, rebounding, and massage therapy.

If they remain swollen, please contact your healthcare provider for further advice.

Flu-like symptoms. This normally occurs in the first week, as your body starts to get rid of bad bacteria. Your body might start to feel tired and achy and you may get a sore throat or runny nose.

This is your immune systems response to your detox. Drink herbal teas with ginger, increase your garlic intake, and take it easy.

Gas and bloating. This is quite common in the first few weeks of the detox plan, particularly if your digestive system has been struggling.

You're also going to be moving more volume and adjusting to new foods, so your small and large intestines will be active.

As bad bacteria leave the body and is replaced by good bacteria, you can experience some temporary gurgling and gas as the body adjusts to increased enzyme productivity.

Make sure you're chewing high fiber foods well, and check you're not eating any foods on the elimination list.

Irritability. If you're a massive coffee drinker or love your sugar, then you could find yourself a little short-tempered in the first week or two.

If you've got a lot of yeast built up, this can cause you to feel irritable as the waste is circulated and eliminated from your system.

You should feel good within two to three days of this showing up, but increase your water intake and try lemon water as well.

Tired. This is quite common in the first week, as an increased metabolic demand on your body increases the amount of energy used, not to mention you're also on a lower calorie intake.

It can take up to five to seven days for your body to adjust, so take it easy and rest when needed.

For more help and troubleshooting ideas, refer to the chapter called *"When Things Go Wrong."*

Honestly, the 28-day *Detox Your Diet* plan is all about self care. Taking care of yourself from the inside out.

You can't go wrong if you increase your water intake and drink herbal teas two to three times a day.

Lemon water is great for dealing with cravings and coffee withdrawal too.

There are specific nutritional products you can also take to help with a lot of these issues, which you can learn more about inside the *Detox Friendly Action Guide,* or by visiting www.detoxyourdietplan.com.

In the next few sections, we'll go into more detail about the detox plan and why we're eliminating the foods we are.

Let's jump straight in.

Foods to Avoid & Foods to Eat

You're probably wondering what exact foods you should be removing from your diet for the next 28 days... Below is a list of all the foods you should avoid, and their suggested replacements.

Foods to Avoid	Foods to Eat
Dairy	Almond, Coconut, Rice & Flax Milk
Gluten/Wheat	Brown Rice, Coconut Flour, Almond Meal
Soy	Raw Almonds
Peanuts & Peanut Butter	Almond Butter
Sugar, Honey, Maple Syrup	Coconut Sugar
Artificial Sweeteners	Stevia, Xylitol
Coffee	Green & Herbal Teas
Alcohol	Non Starchy Vegetables

All Fruit EXCEPT limes, lemons, green apples & berries	Organic green apples & berries
Pork	Cage-Free Eggs
Farm-Raised Fish	Cold Water Fish (limit 1 x per week)
Cage Eggs	Free-Range Chicken & Turkey
All Beef	Grass-Fed Beef
White Potatoes	Sweet Potatoes, Yams, Turnips
Corn	Legumes
Nitrates	Avocado
MSG, Vinegar	Olive Oil, Grapeseed Oil, Coconut Oil, Flaxseed Oil, Apple Cider Vinegar

You'll find a printable version inside the action guide.

On the next few pages, you'll learn why these foods are considered "bad" for us and what they do to our bodies.

And while you might be freaking out about giving

up your favorite foods and dishes, just know that you can generally replicate something similar using healthier options.

Once you understand how the main four foods (gluten, sugar, dairy, and soy) affect your digestive system, you'll find it difficult to go back to eating this stuff. At least that was my experience.

Knowledge is power.

But this isn't a diet. This is not some fad, radical way of living your life.

If you find after your 28-day detox that you want to eat those foods again, then you can!

But you won't...trust me.

Why Gluten-Free?

Are you curious about why gluten and wheat are excluded during the 28-day detox?

There are a couple of reasons, and I'm sure you've heard them before.

Because with the likes of books like *Wheat Belly* by Dr. William Davis and hundreds of thousands of people suffering from Celiac's Disease, a lot of this information is now common knowledge.

But here's some information, just in case you've missed something or you want to refresh your memory.

Did you know it's believed that at least 50% of the US's population has some level of gluten intolerance? That's a very high number.

And for those of you who have suffered from tummy issues, or excess weight around the middle, have you ever considered that wheat-based foods are a large component in causing that?

I've always had tummy issues, whether it was bloating, feeling yucky after a meal — I can't remember the last time I didn't have some type of stomach issue.

But I don't have IBS (I've been tested several times) and apparently, I'm also not gluten-intolerant.

So what's the issue?

Wheat. At least the modern wheat we have access to today. If you haven't read *Wheat Belly* by Dr. William Davis, you should definitely watch this video series where Dr. Oz interviews Dr. Davis about his book and the effects of modern day wheat. You can watch it here: http://www.doctoroz.com/episode/are-you-addicted-wheat?video_id=1998443673001

Unfortunately, the wheat we have access to today has been severely, genetically modified. So much so that it doesn't even closely resemble what our grandmothers had access to back in the 1950s.

Our modern wheat has special properties that make it easily absorbable into our bloodstream, as well as jumping onto our appetite brain receptors to tell us we're more hungrier!

In Dr. Davis's book, and in the video interview with Dr. Oz, he says that two slices of whole wheat bread can increase your blood sugar levels more than a candy bar. To me, that's crazy.

During the next 28 days, take note of how your tummy feels each week that you're NOT consuming wheat or gluten.

Note how much energy you have, how you're sleeping, and how you feel in general.

I can promise you this: You won't feel worse!

Before we move onto sugar, let's talk about food cravings, as you're likely to encounter this during the 28-day detox.

There is no single explanation for food cravings, but they can be caused by the following:

#1: Foods that are HIGH in fats, carbs, and glucose (chocolate, sweets, etc.). These affect your appetite brain receptors, producing endorphins and interactions with the opioid system, which trigger an addictive effect.

For instance, if you're eating foods high in glucose, you'll feel the urge to consume more glucose. This is because the brain has now been conditioned to release "happy hormones" every time you eat glucose.

Your brain is physically changing when it gets used to consuming a large quantity of a certain chemical so it can then release the highest quantity of "happy hormones."

If you think you're an emotional eater...you're not. It's just your brain telling you it wants more of those "happy hormones!"

#2: If your diet consists of foods that aren't considered CLEAN (foods that provide good nutrients and fuel to your body), your body remains "unsatisfied," which can lead to cravings for the "fuel" that is still needed, even though you may have eaten a large amount of food.

I wanted to share these with you because it proves that food cravings are real and that they cause true physical responses in your body, which affects how you eat. YOU are not "mental!" You're also not weak.

Your body is simply responding to the foods you're eating.

This doesn't release you from the responsibility of doing something about your health though. But you can now understand why this is happening and now make steps toward better, healthier choices in your life.

Part of the purpose of doing this 28-day detox is to retrain your brain to crave HEALTHY foods.

If you stick to the plan, you WILL remove those cravings for those addictive, bad foods.

The key is to stick with it long enough to make the physical change happen in your brain.

Ok, let's learn more about sugar...refined sugar that is.

Why Sugar-Free?

As a child, I grew up with my mom's home baked cooking as well as having dessert after dinner every single night.

I'm 100% certain this is why I have such a big sweet tooth...that is, until I did this 28-Day Detox Plan.

Now, I no longer have sweet cravings and instead, prefer healthy options like fruit, to get my 'sweet' fix.

If there's one thing you need to do for your health, it's to ditch refined or processed sugar.

There are a lot of diets out there that will tell you that ALL sugar is bad, and while sugar IS bad, there are some sugars you can incorporate into a healthy lifestyle that won't do to you what refined sugar does....

Let's start by looking at how addictive refined sugar is.

If you haven't seen this enlightening video about how addictive sugar is, then you need to watch it first: https://youtu.be/GljwL4KbLTo

What doesn't seem to be communicated in mainstream media and information in our schools is just how destructive sugar can be on the human body.

Did you know refined sugar can damage, alter, and disrupt proper function of your:

- Nervous system;
- Endocrine system;
- Metabolic system;
- Cardiovascular system;
- Gastrointestinal system; and
- Immune system?

It can also damage, alter, and disrupt primary organs like the liver, kidneys, colon, and pancreas.

And that's just for starters. There is also a large list of health problems directly associated with sugar, which is so enormous that it would take up the rest of this book.

Instead, here's a list of some of the more common problems you might be familiar with:

- Depression, mood swings, aggression, and irritability
- Depletion of mineral levels
- Hyperactivity, anxiety, or panic attacks
- Type 2 diabetes, hypoglycaemia, obesity
- Candida (yeast) overgrowth
- High cholesterol, high blood pressure, heart disease
- Anti-social behavior such as that found in crime and delinquency anger control issues
- Insomnia
- Decreased immune function
- Acne, PMS, OCD, ADD
- Fibromyalgia
- Cancer
- Binging, obesity, addiction
- Chronic fatigue
- Hormone imbalance

Remember, this list is just a dip in the pool when it comes to the health problems an addiction to sugar can cause.

Did you know that the consumption of sugar is considered to be one of the three major causes of degenerative disease in America by the American Diabetes Association?

Doesn't that blow your mind? Doesn't that make you stop and think about what you're putting into your body?

I know it certainly did for me when I read it. Giving up sugar was one of the hardest things I've had to do, but I'd rather experience one to two weeks of headaches, moodiness, and feeling flat than a lifetime of all of those health problems, wouldn't you?

Sugar is so destructive it can be linked to just about any health condition you can think of.

I don't want to go on and on about how bad refined sugar is for you; if you haven't gotten the gist by now, no amount of facts will sway you!

I just want to finish with this:

Removing sugar from your diet is not as easy as you think. Sugar is used as an additive for preservation and to make things more palatable, so it's found in most commercial foods you'll find easily available at your local supermarket.

Unless you are living a health-conscious lifestyle and picking your food wisely, you're going to find sugar is in your ketchup, morning cereal, spaghetti sauce, soup, salad dressing, peanut butter, pancake syrup, bread, yogurt, etc.

You name it, and it probably has sugar in it. They even put sugar in your salt!

The best way to avoid refined sugar is to make food yourself and learn to read labels very carefully.

Sugar may be the hardest thing for you to give up on this 28-day detox, but let me tell you, by week three, you'll start to feel AH-MAZ-ING!

To help fight your sugar cravings, make sure you download the *Detox Friendly Action Guide* (available here: www.detoxyourdietplan.com/free-gift) so you can access all the delicious smoothie recipes!

All healthy and sugar-free, of course.

Why Dairy-Free?

You might be a bit confused about why dairy is on the "avoids" list, but here's some information that will make you think a little differently.

Did you know that pasteurized milk is frequently associated with a worsening of health?

It's crazy to think this, but the Weston Price Foundation states, *"Pasteurization destroys enzymes, diminishes vitamin content, denatures fragile milk proteins, destroys vitamin B12 and vitamin B6, kills beneficial bacteria, promotes pathogens, and is associated with allergies."*

If you live on a farm and can access milk and milk

products that haven't been pasteurized, then this milk is ok to drink.

Pasteurized milk is not real milk. If you have a cup of milk, only 30% of the calcium will be absorbed by your body.

You can actually get twice as much calcium in a cup of broccoli. In fact, many green leafy vegetables have more calcium than a cup of milk.

I know which I'd prefer to consume.

The other thing about milk is that it is high in milk sugar and lactose, which can cause allergic reactions in some people.

The reason we use an "avoids" list on the 28-day detox is to remove all potential issues arising, particularly if you're like me and have had some tummy issues for a while but have never been able to figure out why.

By removing dairy from your diet for the next 28 days, you allow your body to breathe and reset, then you can see if you have issues with dairy when you reintroduce it back in.

You should also consider where your milk is coming from. Unless it's certified organic, for all you know, the milk you're drinking has come from a dairy cow that has been given growth hormones.

Growth hormones can increase the risk of certain diseases or even hormonal imbalances.

So even after the 28-day detox, you should only consume organic milk and milk-based products, if you choose to do so at all.

Personally, I much prefer almond and coconut milks, because I NEVER experience an upset tummy from either of them.

This is why it's important to monitor and track your 28-day detox progress, which we'll talk about shortly.

Why Soy and Corn-Free?

To be honest, when I started this plan, I was surprised that corn and soy were on the "avoids" list too.

I mean, corn is so yummy and healthy, right? And soy, I only use that when I'm cooking Asian-inspired dishes; how harmful could that be?

Corn

Similar to wheat, the corn we have access to today has been severely modified and changed due to the high demand for the consumption of corn world-wide.

This has led to hormone modifications to the point that corn can now cause just as many issues as wheat.

Removing corn from your diet for the next 28 days will allow your body to reset, and if you want to eat corn after this time, opt for organic and in-season options only.

Soy

Phytoestrogens in soy can mimic the effects of the female hormone estrogen. These can cause adverse effects on various human tissues.

For example, if you were to drink two glasses of soy milk a day for 30 days, you would have consumed enough of the chemical to alter your menstrual cycle.

Side note: Soy lecithin doesn't have the same effect and is safe to consume.

Now that we've covered the main reasons for avoiding these foods, let's jump into the next section where we're going to talk about how important it is to track and measure your progress, including keeping a daily food journal.

Jump into the next section to get started.

Track & Measure

To understand whether you've been successful with the detox plan, you need to measure and chart your progress.

To measure, you need to track. To track, you need to know why you're doing this!

Basically, before you get started, you want to make sure you know what your end-goal for doing the detox is.

If you want to feel healthier, write that down. If you want to have more energy and feel good from the inside out, write that down. If you want to lose weight and make healthier food choices, write that down.

If it's all of the above, write it down!

Inside the action guide, you'll find a fillable sheet where you can write down your reasons for doing the detox. Make sure you fill that out and refer back to it when you're in struggle-town.

Measure Your Progress

Now that you know why you're doing this, you need to take all your measurements so you can track your progress.

Start with weighing yourself.

You'll only do this twice, once at the beginning and once at the end.

Avoid weighing yourself during the next 28 days, as the scales don't always tell the truth!

Take a "before" picture. You don't have to share it with anyone; this is purely for your benefit.

Take measurements around your chest, bicep, waist, hips, and thigh.

You only need to do this on one side, so opt for the right side if you're right-handed, left side if you're left-handed.

Not sure where to measure? Check out the image below and then note down in the action guide your Day 1 measurements.

Each week, take your measurements. Make sure to do it at the same time on the same day each week, so you're able to compare apples with apples.

The image on the next page gives you a rough idea of where to measure. You'll find printable pages inside your *Detox Friendly Action Guide* too.

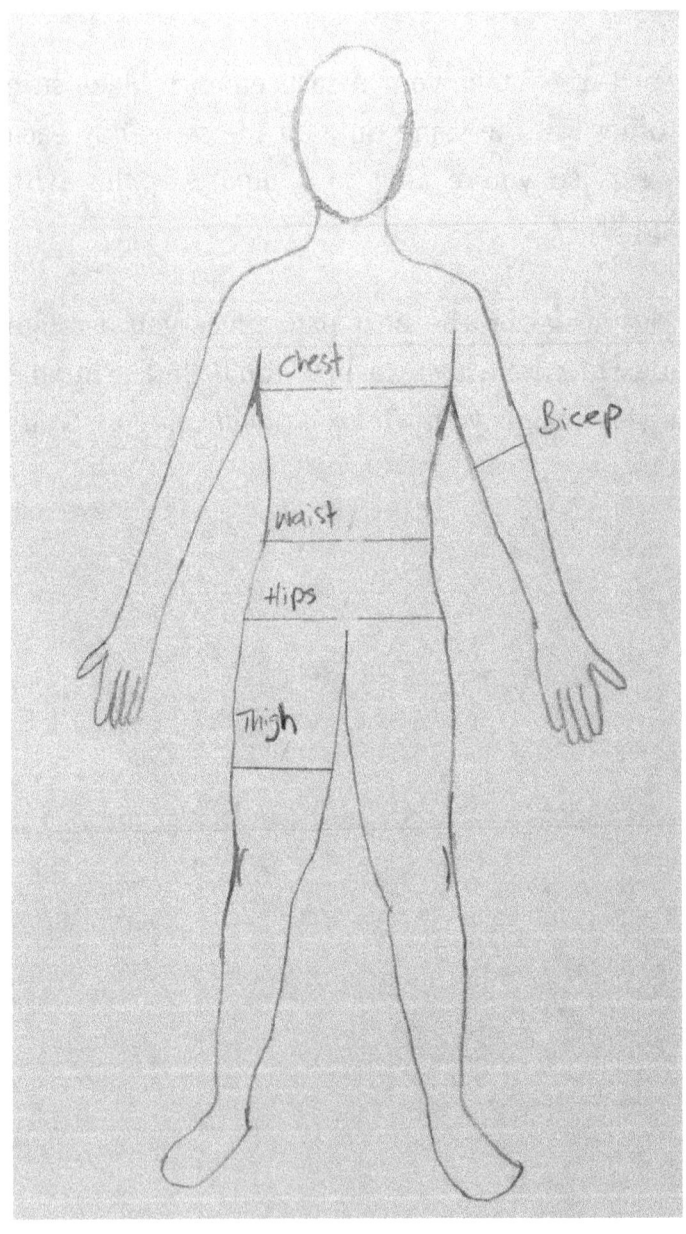

Track Your Results

Using the space inside the action guide, enter your measurements each week. As the weeks go by, you'll be able to track your results and see your progress.

On the last day of the detox, weigh yourself, but also note how your clothes feel and how you look.

Take your "after" picture and compare it with your before.

You should be able to see a noticeable difference if you were following the weight loss plan.

If you were solely detoxing, you should notice a flatter tummy and some weight loss.

Don't forget to do this.

You can't see where you started or how far you've come without some data.

And if you continue to do another 28 days, this will be important to help track your ongoing progress.

Daily Food Journal

As well as tracking your physical measurements, it's important to track what you're eating and how you're feeling.

Below is a sample journal page. You can use this format and create your own journal (a blank notebook is perfect for this), or you could print off the journal page from inside the *Detox Friendly Action Guide* 28 times and record your food intake that way.

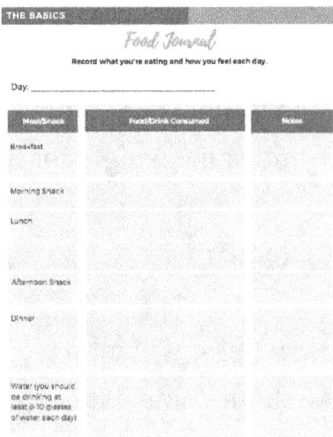

Another alternative is to use a note-taking app

like Evernote or the notes app on your smartphone, whatever works best for you.

If you'd prefer to take photos of your food and track things that way, do that too.

I find that by writing down everything I eat each day, including how much water I've consumed, I can better monitor any foods that make me feel yuck.

It makes it a lot easier to figure out and troubleshoot solutions if you're tracking what you're eating.

In the next section, you can check out the plans and get started on your own 28-Day *Detox Your Diet* plan!

Week-by-Week Plans

Below are a couple of plans for you to follow, depending on what your goals are for the end of the detox.

As long as you follow what is outlined for you and stick to the basics of the plan, you will achieve your health-related goals. It can take two to three repeats to achieve your optimal weight, so don't be discouraged if you don't lose all the weight you want in the first 28 days.

In fact, it would be extremely unhealthy to expect to lose 15kgs in 28 days. Instead, what's normal is between 3-5kgs every 28 days.

Plan 1: Detox + Weight Loss

WEEK 1
- Start the day with a detox tea (this should be herbal).
- Aim to have breakfast at least 13 hours after your last meal the night before (aim to eat dinner no later than 7pm and

breakfast no earlier than 8am). Have a shake for breakfast made from water or almond milk with a pea/rice protein, good fat, and berries.

- Have a snack around mid-morning. Options include a green apple with almond butter or avocado and brown rice crackers.
- Lunch should be another shake. Make sure you've drunk at least half of your daily water intake by now (4-5 glasses).
- Dinner should be a clean, whole food meal based on the portion sizes shown in the plan under Step 2: Replace.
- End the day with another detox tea.
- Add 30 minutes of exercise from Day 4.
- Repeat this eating plan for the next 7 days.

WEEK 2

- The same as Week 1 above but increasing exercise if you can.
- Repeat for the next 7 days.

WEEK 3

- Stop drinking the detox tea and instead, drink a cleanse tea throughout the day.

> This should be brewed and drunk cold, slowly throughout the day.

- Breakfast, snack, lunch, and dinner remain the same.
- You might choose to drop your exercising this week or reduce it to low-impact, depending on how you feel.
- Repeat this cleanse week for 7 days.

WEEK 4

- The same as Week 1 & 2, making sure you're drinking enough water and tracking your measurements.

Plan 2: Detox Only

WEEK 1
- Start the day with a detox tea (this should be herbal).
- Aim to have breakfast at least 13 hours after your last meal the night before (aim to eat dinner no later than 7pm and breakfast no earlier than 8am). Have a shake for breakfast made from water or almond milk with a pea/rice protein, good fat, and berries.
- Have a snack around mid-morning. Options include green apple with almond butter or avocado and brown rice crackers.
- Lunch should be a clean, whole food meal. Make sure you've drunk at least half of your daily water intake by now (4-5 glasses).
- Dinner should be a smaller clean, whole food meal based on the portion sizes shown in the plan under Step 2: Replace.
- End the day with another detox tea.
- Add 30 minutes of exercise from Day 4.
- Repeat this eating plan for the next 7 days.

WEEK 2

- The same as Week 1 above but increasing exercise if you can.
- Repeat for the next 7 days.

WEEK 3

- Stop drinking the detox tea and instead, drink a cleanse tea throughout the day. This should be brewed and drunk cold, slowly throughout the day.
- Breakfast, snack, lunch and dinner remain the same.
- You might choose to drop your exercising this week or reduce it to low-impact, depending on how you feel.
- Repeat this cleanse week for 7 days.

WEEK 4

- The same as Week 1 & 2, making sure you're drinking enough water and tracking your measurements.

Sample Meal Plans

Sample Meal Plan (Weight Loss):

7:00am Wakeup:

Detox tea (choose one of the following options)
Arbonne Essentials Herbal Tea (refer to the *Recommended Nutritional Products* page for details)
Organic green tea

8:30am Breakfast:

Strawberry, Mint & Cucumber Shake

- 1 cup fresh (or frozen) organic strawberries, chopped
- 1/2 cup organic Persian cucumber
- 2 leaves fresh organic mint
- 2 scoops Arbonne vanilla pea/rice protein powder (NO WHEY! Refer to *Recommended Nutritional Products* page for details)
- 4 oz water
- 1 cup coconut milk
- Ice cubes

Blend!

10:30am Snack:
Options
- Berries & coconut milk
- Green apple & 1 tsp almond butter
- 1/2 avocado & 2 brown rice crackers

12:30pm Lunch:
Chocolate Almond Delight Shake
- 12 oz unsweetened almond milk
- 15 raw almonds (or 1 tsp almond butter)
- 1/2 tsp coconut extract
- 1 Tbsp cacao nibs
- 2 scoops Arbonne chocolate pea/rice protein powder (NO WHEY! Refer to *Recommended Nutritional Products* page for details)
- 6 ice cubes

Blend until smooth!

4:30pm Snack:
Options
- Berries & coconut milk
- Green apple & 1 tsp almond butter

- 1/2 avocado & 2 brown rice crackers

5:30pm Dinner:
Avocado Pasta

- 2 Tbsps sea salt (for pasta)
- 1 pound brown rice pasta
- 2 ripe avocados
- 2 Tbsps lemon juice
- 3 large cloves garlic
- 3/4 cup fresh basil leaves
- 2 Tsps sea salt
- 1/2 tsp ground black pepper
- 1/4 cup extra virgin olive oil
- Vegetable mix ins (optional)
  - 1 cup frozen peas
  - 1/2 cup cherry tomatoes
  - 1/2 cup roasted red peppers
  - 1/2 cup frozen broccoli, steamed

Instructions

Bring a large pot of salted water to boil. Add pasta and cook according to packet directions.

While the pasta boils, throw the avocado, lemon juice, garlic, basil leaves, salt, and pepper into a food processor or blender. Blend until smooth.

Once the pasta is ready, drain it and return to the pot. Add in the avocado mixture and stir to mix. Drizzle in olive oil and add any vegetables you want.

Stir to combine and top with basil if desired.

Found at http://tiphero.com/avocado-pasta

8:00pm Detox Tea
Options
Arbonne Essentials Herbal Tea
Organic green tea

Sample Meal Plan (Detox Only):

7:00am Wakeup:
Detox tea
Arbonne Essentials Herbal Tea
Organic green tea

8:30am Breakfast:
Strawberry, Mint & Cucumber Shake

- 1 cup fresh (or frozen) organic strawberries, chopped
- 1/2 cup organic Persian cucumber
- 2 leaves fresh organic mint
- 2 scoops Arbonne vanilla pea/rice protein powder (NO WHEY! Refer to *Recommended Nutritional Products* page for details)
- 4 oz water
- 1 cup coconut milk
- Ice cubes

Blend!

10:30am Snack:
Options
- Berries & coconut milk
- Green apple & 1 tsp almond butter
- 1/2 avocado & 2 brown rice crackers

12:30pm Lunch:
Cucumber Salad with Lime & Cilantro
- 1 small red onion, sliced
- 2 cucumbers, peeled or sliced
- 3 medium limes, juiced
- 2 Tbsp cilantro, finely chopped

- 2 Tbsp extra virgin olive oil
- Sea salt
- Black pepper

Instructions

Place the sliced cucumbers, sliced onion, lime juice, chopped cilantro, and olive oil in a bowl.

Mix well. Taste and add sea salt as needed.

Serve immediately or let rest refrigerated for at least 30 minutes before eating.

Pair with cold-water fish or free-range chicken (optional).

4:30pm Snack:
Options
- Berries & coconut milk
- Green apple & 1 tsp almond butter
- 1/2 avocado & 2 brown rice crackers

5:30pm Dinner:
Avocado Pasta
- 2 Tbsps sea salt (for pasta)
- 1 pound brown rice pasta

- 2 ripe avocados
- 2 Tbsps lemon juice
- 3 large cloves garlic
- 3/4 cup fresh basil leaves
- 2 tsps sea salt
- 1/2 tsp ground black pepper
- 1/4 cup extra virgin olive oil
- Vegetable mix ins (optional)
    - 1 cup frozen peas
    - 1/2 cup cherry tomatoes
    - 1/2 cup roasted red peppers
    - 1/2 cup frozen broccoli, steamed

Instructions

Bring a large pot of salted water to boil. Add pasta and cook according to packet directions.

While the pasta boils, throw the avocado, lemon juice, garlic, basil leaves, salt, and pepper into a food processor or blender. Blend until smooth.

Once the pasta is ready, drain it and return to the pot. Add in the avocado mixture and stir to mix. Drizzle olive oil and add any vegetables you want.

Stir to combine and top with basil if desired.

Found at http://tiphero.com/avocado-pasta

8:00pm Detox Tea
Options
Arbonne Essentials Herbal Tea
Organic green tea

For a range of clean-eating recipes, refer to the *Detox Friendly Action Guide* here: www.detoxyourdietplan.com/free-gift

What to Do When Things Go Wrong

You are unique. I am unique. No two people are the same, so it stands to reason that the experience you'll have during the 28-Day Detox Plan will be different from another person taking it at the same time.

It also makes sense that you are likely to run into a few challenges, particularly if you've been eating a diet that largely consists of most of the "foods to avoid."

As I've already highlighted in the *"What to Expect"* section of the **Detox Your Diet** plan, there are some common things you may experience, particularly in the first week of the detox.

Here they are again:

- Severe headaches
- Constipation and/or diarrhoea
- Strong body odor
- Swollen lymph nodes

- Flu-like symptoms
- Gas and bloating
- Feeling irritable
- Tired and exhausted

But what about other issues? What about things that might crop up during the detox that are outside of these issues?

Read the frequently asked questions and answers below to help "troubleshoot" your own special circumstances.

If you can't find the answer, come and join the private Facebook group to get additional support here: https://www.facebook.com/groups/1462896360429941/

Frequently Asked Questions & Answers

Q: I'm feeling really tired and fatigued. What can I do?

A: If you're in the first week of the detox, this is normal. Avoid any exercise for the first three to five days and LISTEN to your body. By day five you should be feeling good again.

If you're still feeling this way after day five, then review your shakes and snacks. You need to make sure you're still eating good fats and carbs at your one meal as well.

Seek medical advice if you're still feeling tired for longer than seven days.

Q: I'm feeling a big "slump" in the afternoon, is this because of my coffee addiction?!

A: Absolutely! It could also be from your sugar addiction. To combat this, drink more water and herbal tea, or check out the recommended nutritional products (inside the action guide) for ideas on what supplements you can take to combat this.

But bottom line, keep hydrated.

Q: I'm experiencing pain in my stomach and joints; what's going on?

A: This is a common withdrawal symptom of coffee and black tea. It generally subsides after three to four days.

This is the time it takes for receptors in the brain to get rid of caffeine consumption. Drink more herbal or detox tea to help. You can also switch to decaffeinated beverages.

Q: I am craving carbs! I miss my sugary cakes and bread. I'm constantly hungry and irritable.

A: These symptoms mean your body is starting to use your fat stores. This process is called ketosis and is EXACTLY what you want to happen.

If you're feeling hungry, drink lemon with water and make sure you're including good fats in your shakes. Remember, you still have to eat!

Q: I've decided to do the vegetarian version of the detox, but I'm not sure what to expect.

A: Red meat can cause the body to have a high acidity level. Removing meat from your diet will allow the body to return to a healthier alkaline state.

Doing this encourages the body to get rid of the acid, through your pores, which can leave behind a strong odor, foul breath, and a bitter taste in your mouth.

Once all the acid has disappeared from your body, these symptoms will disappear.

To combat the withdrawals, consume a lot of fruit, vegetables, and lemon water.

Q: I've noticed that I'm quite lethargic and have mood swings. Why is this?

A: Aside from your body going into withdrawal from a lot of foods, these specific symptoms are common when we eliminate dairy food from our diet.

You might struggle to sleep, become lethargic and groggy, and experience mood swings, headaches, and potentially constipation.

Drink coconut or almond milk and their products instead. Your symptoms will disappear once your body is rid of the bad bacteria caused by dairy products.

Q: I am absolutely CRAVING sugar and sugar products! I feel low on energy too. What can I do?

A: Sugar withdrawals are similar to those you might experience with drugs or alcohol.

If you are experiencing severe sugar withdrawals, start removing sugar slowly, rather than going cold turkey.

Replace it with coconut sugar, as well as fresh, seasonal (organic) fruits, salads, and almonds.

Q: I recently had my period and now I'm experiencing another one! Is this normal?

A: Some woman, particularly those on the contraceptive pill, may find an unscheduled period happens during their detox.

This isn't a normal period, but rather part of the body's detoxing process.

There is nothing you can do to stop it. Take good care of yourself and continue to drink a lot of lemon water and herbal teas. Your "period" should stop within five to seven days.

If your period continues past the seven-day mark, stop drinking any herbal teas, as these can also bring on a "detox period." Once your period stops, slowly reintroduce your herbal teas.

Seek medical advice if you're unsure.

Q: I am going through menopause but have just started to notice spotting and a few stomach cramps here and there. What's going on?

A: A detox is a great option if you're going through menopause. It can help decrease menopausal symptoms and helps clean out the liver to help it regenerate, reducing the risk of cancer and other serious illnesses.

Some women may experience a light period during this detox. This is perfectly normal and is just your body's detox system cleaning everything out.

The spotting or light bleeding should stop within seven days. If it doesn't, please seek medical advice from your doctor.

Q: I'm feeling bloated all the time. It's really uncomfortable and discouraging to feel this way. What's happening?

A: Bloating is a common side effect of good bacteria starting to grow and bad bacteria leaving your body. It can also happen if you're not used to having a lot of fiber in your diet.

If you find yourself bloating a lot after the first week of the detox plan, look to reduce the amount of fiber you're having each day, aiming to have about half of the fiber you were eating.

Slowly increase the amount of fiber you're eating and make sure you're drinking a LOT of water to help flush out your system.

Fiber is important to your detox — it's what helps move the bad bacteria and fat out of your body.

Q: I've just weighed and measured myself and I've gained weight; help!

A: This is quite normal throughout the 28 days of the detox. It's quite common to gain weight in the first week, as you're likely retaining more water and bloating.

Continue doing what you're doing and stick with the detox plan. You will lose weight.

Watch what you're putting in your shakes and what you're eating for your whole clean meal. Stick to the serving suggestions and portion sizes.

Also know that one day of "falling off the wagon" can undo three to five days of good eating. That's all it takes for bad bacteria to set up shop in your system.

Make sure you're incorporating at least three days a week of high intensity exercise as well. If this is difficult to do, at least go for a walk each day for 30 minutes.

This will help stimulate your digestive system and

eliminate toxins and fat faster.

At-Home Exercise Options

While exercising during the detox isn't compulsory, it will help you to eliminate those toxic foods faster.

Movement stimulates your digestive system, which is exactly what we want. A stimulated digestive system works optimally to remove bad bacteria from your body.

As mentioned, during the first three to five days of the detox, you'll want to either not exercise or do low-impact workouts.

If you're completely new to exercising at home, or haven't exercised regularly in over three months, you'll want to take things slow.

In my book *No Gym Needed*, I talk about lots of different exercises you can do at home without gym equipment or special machines. You can pick up your own copy on Amazon here: http://amzn.to/2lRtKTn.

The best exercise routines that will support the

detox plan include HIIT (high intensity workouts), Tabata, and circuit-type workouts.

You should aim to do these for 30-60 minutes, three to four times per week.

Below you'll find some workouts to get you started.

HIIT Number 1

This workout will get the heart pumping and should take you approximately 15-20 minutes, once you've mastered the moves. This is the perfect workout for a beginner.

If you're intermediate or advanced, you can repeat this 2-3 times for an extra cardio workout.

Warmup:

    20 jumping jacks

    :30 sec high knees

    :30 sec butt kicks

    5 jump squats

:15 second water BREAK

Workout:

    :40 sec mountain climbers
     5 burpees
     30 jumping jacks
    :40 sec jump rope
    (Pro Hack: no jump rope necessary, just pretend you're actually doing the motion!)
     5 jump squats
    :30 sec BREAK

    :40 sec march in place
    :20 sec high knees
    :20 sec butt kickers
    :15 sec water break
     40 jumping jacks
    :50 sec jump rope
    5 burpees
    :30 sec BREAK

    :45 sec run in place
    :30 sec water break
     30 jumping jacks
     10 jump squats
     5 burpees
    :30 sec BREAK

:30 sec jump rope

5 squats

:30 sec water break

20 jumping jacks

:25 sec high knees

5 squats

5 burpees

:30 sec march

HIIT Number 2

This 20-minute workout will have you sweating. This is the workout I use when I'm travelling or don't have a lot of room to move around.

Warmup:

20 jumping jacks

:30 sec high knees

:30 sec butt kickers

5 jump squats

Workout:

:30 sec side lunges

:60 sec jumping jacks

:30 sec squats

:60 sec jog in place

:30 sec burpees

:60 sec jump rope

:30 sec lunges

:60 sec butt kickers

:30 sec BREAK

:30 sec mountain climbers

:60 sec march in place

:30 sec speed skaters

:60 sec jumping jacks

:30 sec side lunges

:30 sec push ups

:30 sec water break

Repeat 2 times. Rest for 1 minute before repeating.

Tabata Workout

- Jumping jacks - 20 seconds, rest for 10 seconds

- Alternating backward lunge (step backwards each lunge rather than forwards) - 20 seconds, rest for 10 seconds

- Plank - 20 seconds, rest for 10 seconds
- Sit-ups/crunches - 20 seconds, rest for 10 seconds

Repeat twice, then rest for 60 seconds.

Do this 5-10 times for a great workout.

You'll find more options inside the action guide too.

What's Next?

Congratulations! You've completed the 28-Day *Detox Your Diet* plan!

How are you feeling?

I'd love to hear how you did. If you're open to sharing your story and photos, I'd welcome the opportunity to chat with you via email. You can share your story with me by sending an email to lise@lisecartwright.com.

Now that you've finished, you might be wondering "What happens next?"

There are a number of options for you.

Option 1: Repeat Another 28-Day Detox

If, like me, you have had years of eating a lot of the bad foods and want to make sure you're fully detoxed, you simply repeat the detox plan again.

Do everything the same, including making sure to track your meals, even if you "cheat" — it's important to keep track of what you're eating so you can make note of any changes in your body.

Option 2: Add Back Avoid Foods

If you're happy with how the detox went for you and you're ready to get back to a "normal" eating routine, it's time to add back in the "avoid" foods.

BUT, make sure you read the following before you do this, as there is a system to follow to do this right.

You don't want to add everything back all at once, as this can send your body into a meltdown and all those problems you had pre-detox are more than likely to come rushing back.

Instead, follow these steps:

Step 1: Introduce soy back into your diet. Start by drinking a glass of soy milk and note how you feel 30 minutes to an hour later.

Weigh and measure yourself the next morning to see if you've gained any weight overnight.

Your body reacts to allergenic foods by filling your tissues with water, which is why you gain weight.

Do this for three consecutive days.

If you do see weight gain and/or any bloating, gas, etc, then it's likely you have a sensitivity to soy or may be allergic.

Solution: Remove soy from your diet permanently.

Step 2: Introduce corn back into your diet. Start by eating a meal with corn in it and note how you feel 30 minutes to an hour later.

Weigh and measure yourself the next morning to see if you've gained any weight overnight.

Do this for three consecutive days.

If you do see weight gain and/or any bloating, gas, etc, then it's likely you have a sensitivity to corn or may be allergic.

Solution: Remove corn from your diet

permanently.

Step 3: Introduce dairy back into your diet. Start by drinking a glass of milk followed by eating some cheese and note how you feel 30 minutes to an hour later.

Weigh and measure yourself the next morning to see if you've gained any weight overnight.

Do this for three consecutive days.

If you do see weight gain and/or any bloating, gas, etc, then it's likely you have a sensitivity to dairy or may be allergic.

Solution: Remove dairy from your diet permanently.

Step 4: Introduce refined sugar back into your diet. Start by eating foods that contain a high amount of refined sugar, like sweets and cakes, and note how you feel 30 minutes to an hour later.

Weigh and measure yourself the next morning to

see if you've gained any weight overnight.

Do this for three consecutive days.

If you do see weight gain and/or any bloating, gas, etc, then it's likely you have a sensitivity to refined sugar or may be allergic.

Solution: Remove refined sugar from your diet permanently.

Step 5: Lastly, introduce gluten and wheat back into your diet. Start by eating foods that contain a high amount of gluten and wheat, like breads and pastas, and note how you feel 30 minutes to an hour later.

Weigh and measure yourself the next morning to see if you've gained any weight overnight.

Do this for three consecutive days.

If you do see weight gain and/or any bloating, gas, etc, then it's likely you have a sensitivity to gluten and wheat or may be allergic.

Solution: Remove wheat/gluten from your diet permanently.

Option 3: Maintain a Healthy Eating Lifestyle

If you're happy with eating the *Detox Your Diet* way, you can continue with this type of whole food eating permanently.

It's best to apply the 80/20 rule once you've satisfactorily completed the program to your liking.

The aim is that, for 80% of the time, you'll follow this type of healthy eating plan and 20% of the time, you'll indulge.

This means focusing on eating balanced meals of lean protein, carbohydrates, good fats, and non-starchy vegetables.

If you were able to do it for the past 28 days, it should now be easy to continue eating this way, with a slight modification in that you might choose to eat two whole meals a day, particularly if you're at a weight you'd like to maintain.

If you'd like to continue losing weight, then you can simply continue with the 28-day detox plan.

Remember, this plan is about resetting your diet and body and allowing its natural detox system to function properly.

The more you load it up with the "avoid" foods, the less likely it will be able to deal with them... but if you stick to the 80/20 rule, your body will be able to handle the odd indulgence and detox without any additional help.

Want Even More?

Want faster results? Then you need to look at the vegan line of products mentioned in the "Recommended Nutritional Products" section inside the Action Guide, or visit the website to learn more:

www.detoxyourdietplan.com.

References

#1: Confronting the failure of behavioral and dietary treatments for obesity

By David M. Garner, Michigan State University, USA and
Susan C. Wooley, University of Cincinnati, USA

http://www.sciencedirect.com/science/article/pii/027273589190128H

#2: Dieting does not work

By Traci Mann

www.sciencedaily.com/releases/2007/04/070404162428.htm

#3: Low calorie dieting increases cortisol

By Tomiyama AJ, Mann T, Vinas D, Hunger JM, Dejager J, and Taylor SE.

https://www.ncbi.nlm.nih.gov/pubmed/20368473

Can You Help?

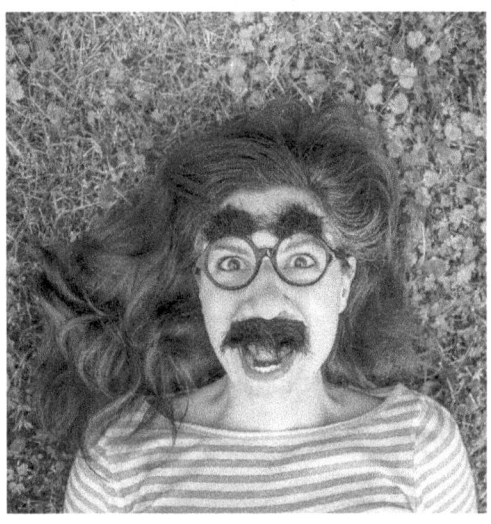

Thanks so much for reading my book. I really appreciate your feedback and I LOVE hearing what you have to say.

So with that in mind, I need your input to make the next version of this book even better.

Please leave a helpful and honest REVIEW on Amazon by visiting Amazon and accessing your purchases to leave your review.

Thanks so much!

~ Lise

About the Author

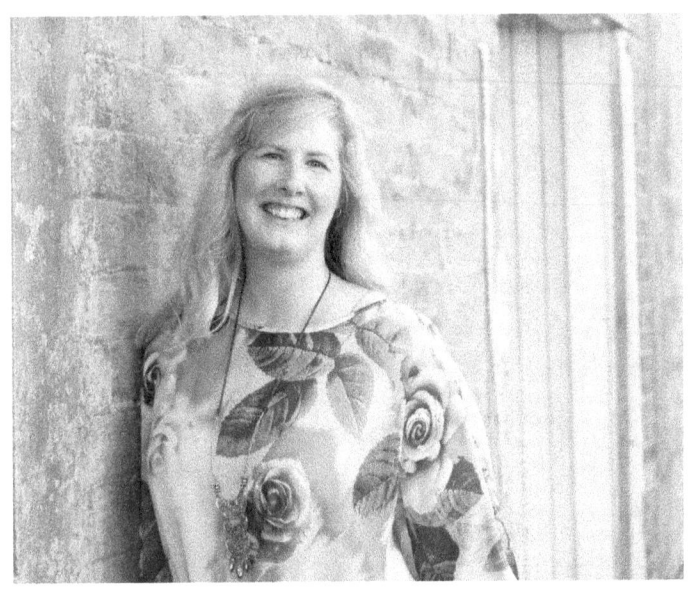

Lise Cartwright

Lise is an author, blogger and sometimes-social media consultant and a self-confessed shoe fanatic – she's obsessed. Just ask her husband!

She has been looking for the magic in life since she was first exposed to positive, happy thoughts at the tender age of one - thanks Mum and Dad!

Lise can regularly be found at local cafes, NOT drinking coffee, but the more sophisticated and magical beverage that is a *Chai Latte*.

If you're looking to connect with Lise, you can stalk her on Facebook, annoy her on Twitter or send her an email.

Her online home is located at hustleandgroove.com.

More Books

Below is a list of the other titles written by Lise Cartwright.

Side Hustle Blueprint: How to Make an Extra $1000 in 30 Days Without Leaving Your Day Job!

Side Hustle Blueprint: How to Make an Extra $1000 per month Writing eBooks!

Outsourced Freelancing Success Series:

- Book 1: Start a Successful Freelancing Business & Make Your First Dollar Online!
- Book 2: How to Set Freelancing Rates and Get Paid What You're Worth
- Book 3: How to Protect Your Freelancing Business With Client Contracts That Work!
- Book 4: How to Set Up and Structure Your Freelancing Business The Right Way
- Book 5: Top 57 Freelancing Job Sites For Finding High Paying, Quality Clients Fast
- Book 6: 101+ Tools, Apps & Programs to

Help You Run a Successful Freelancing Business

- Book 7: 18 Ways to Grow Your Freelancing Business in 30 Days or Less

No Gym Needed: Quick & Simple Workouts for Gals on the Go. Get a Toned Body in 30 Minutes or Less!

COMING SOON:
- ***No Gym Needed:*** *The Beginners Guide to Quick & Simple At-Home Workouts*
- ***More books in the Detox Your [insert focus area here!] series***

If you'd like to get first dibs on new books as they are released, make sure you join the ***Reader's Club*** here:

http://www.hustleandgroove.com/lises-readers-club